Spirituality and Your Health

Reflections of a Pharmacology Teacher

Joseph Leo Borowitz

Copyright © 2019 by Joseph Borowitz

ISBN-10	1642540706
ISBN-13	9781642540703

All rights reserved. No part of this book may be reproduced or transmitted in any form or by any means, electronic or mechanical, including photocopying, recording, or by any information storage and retrieval system, without permission in writing from the copyright owner.

Scripture taken from the New King James Version. Copyright 1979, 1980, 1982 by Thomas Nelson, inc. Used by permission. All rights reserved.

Contents

Acknowledgement 5

Introduction 6

Chapter 1 ..... Our Need for High-Quality Medical Education .. 9

Chapter 2 ..... Some Problems in Medicine Today 15

Chapter 3 ..... What on Earth Are You Doing, for God's Sake? . 25

Chapter 4 ..... The Proper Motivation Is Essential 38

Chapter 5 ..... Divine Healing 44

Chapter 6 ..... Spiritual Warfare 51

Chapter 7 ..... Holy Spirit Power 60

Chapter 8 ..... Importance of Humility 69

Chapter 9 ..... Outstanding Health Personnel 73

Chapter 10 .... Humor and Healing 81

Chapter 11 .... Importance of Fellowship and Teamwork 89

Chapter 12 .... Contributions of Pharmacology to Society 92

Chapter 13 .... A Commentary on Modern Medical Practice ... 98

Chapter 14 .... Divine Healing versus Modern Medicine 105

Chapter 15 .... Importance of Relationships 108

Chapter 16 .... Conclusion 120

Index 125

Acknowledgement

My Pastor at Blessed Sacrament Church in West Lafayette, Indiana during the time this book was written was Father David Buckles. His spiritual direction and guidance are acknowledged. The editorial help of Donald Mitchell, PhD is also acknowledged. He is Professor Emeritus of Religious Studies at Purdue University and serves as Advisor for the US Conference of Catholic Bishops. Don also wrote a review of this book which appears on the back cover.

Introduction

This book is the result of fifty years' effort in medical and pharmacy education. But only in the last thirty years have I added a spiritual, godly aspect to my teaching. It made a real difference. This is also a book of miracles, miracles of healing and personal miracles. So many amazing things have happened to guide me along the way. I've outlined my family background and the story of how I got into this business and also explained how my spiritual experience enhanced my effectiveness as a teacher. The strong relationship between faith, positive hope, and health is emphasized throughout the book.

Most Americans (95 percent) believe in God, and 57 percent pray every day (D. Sulmasy, *The Healer's Calling*, Paulist Press, Mahwah, New Jersey, 1997). Also there is evidence that being involved in organized religion promotes health (Jeff Levin, *God, Faith, and Health*, John Wiley and Sons, New York, NY, 2001). No matter what denomination, if you're an active member, you will live longer on the average than people who don't go to church. There is some health-giving benefit of church membership. This book examines some of the possible reasons for this observation.

Scientific, social, or spiritual factors may be involved in explaining the data. Regardless of the mechanisms, everyone should be aware of the vitality provided by a godly lifestyle.

Physicians and pharmacists are obviously key players in health matters and have a great influence on each of us at critical times in our lives. This book proposes that all medical personnel be thoroughly trained not only in scientific, but also in social and spiritual areas to be maximally effective.

CHAPTER 1

Our Need for High-Quality Medical Education

I cannot pray like Peter. I cannot preach like Paul. But I can tell all the folks in Gilead, there is balm enough for all.
—African-American spiritual

For each of us, our health is a primary aspect of our lives. We think about it every day. Most of us take vitamins, eat well, and exercise to keep ourselves in good shape. When something goes wrong, we can see a physician. This is something we keep in the backs of our minds. We can always get help when we need it. We trust our physicians and expect them to be ready to step in and do their jobs when necessary. We assume they are well-trained, sensible people and have good judgment in health matters and that they will do the best they can for us.

Do we assume too much? I don't think so. I believe a loving God would call honest, capable men and women into the healing ministry to care for us. This presumes God would also call others to be teachers, scientists, nurses, pharmacists, and technicians, etc., to support physicians in their efforts to maintain the health of human beings, the greatest of God's creation. All these people working together and doing their level best should make us feel secure in health matters. If we ever need help, we can have access to the finest of treatments.

I was walking between the pharmacy and nursing buildings at Purdue one day last winter. It was cold, and there was snow on the ground. There on a branch of a ginkgo tree sat a squirrel making the most mournful, low screeching sound I ever heard. Its tail was curved up over its back. It was obviously not feeling well and was complaining. My heart went out to it, but there was nothing I could do except say a little prayer. God created wild animals and provides for them, but they don't have a network of health-care providers that we humans do. We should be grateful for our many blessings.

When I was in graduate school at Northwestern, I took courses with the medical students. They were stiff competition. They worked all the time. You could find them there studying almost anytime in the evenings or on weekends. There was so much to learn in such a short time. The work ethic of medical students has not changed through the years. They still want to be good physicians and to excel in their studies and prepare themselves to be of greatest possible service to us in our needs.

So medical students still have high hopes and medical education in this country is good and we in the United States depend on it. We all feel more secure knowing that there are dedicated people available to help us when we have health problems. The system is not always perfect, but thank God for these talented, good-hearted professionals. They undergird the structure of our hectic lifestyles and provide a safety net to catch us if we fall. Quality education of medical personnel is of utmost importance in the United States today.

Most of us have deep-seated ideals that drive us on and make life more worthwhile. Many people love their spouses and families and are willing to do anything to improve their home life. Others are eager to excel at their work, to do a really good job that will benefit their companies or their communities. Some want to win that Nobel Prize or to make some other lasting contribution to society. Still others are devoted to building God's kingdom here on earth and to bring justice with its resulting peace into reality. Those in the health professions prepare themselves to look after the welfare of others, to allow us to live full life spans with body and mind still fully functional.

The Hippocratic oath not only is a standard for professional medical practice, but also provides quality assurance for us as potential patients. It is attributed to Hippocrates, a Greek physician born in the year 460. It is sometimes sworn to by new physicians and may be incorporated into graduation ceremonies of medical colleges. It states that "physicians will prescribe regimens for the good of their patients according to their ability and never do harm to anyone. They will not give a lethal drug to anyone if asked and will not give a woman a pessary to cause an abortion. But they will preserve the purity of their own lives and their arts. They will have in mind only the good of their patients, keeping themselves from all intentional ill-doing and all seduction. All that may come to their knowledge in the exercise of their profession or in daily commerce with men and which ought not to be spread abroad, they will keep secret and will never reveal." The sentiments of the oath of Hippocrates are not just lofty altruism but, for many physicians, a genuine desire to serve as a mediator for God to restore health and function to human beings. These simple ethical principles are a motivating, guiding force of the practice of medicine and are truths that we rely on when seeking medical help.

The godly call to serve people as pharmacists is just as serious as that for doctors. Pharmacists are important, well-respected members of their communities. Our Christian Pharmacy Student Association at Purdue came up with "oath of a Christian pharmacist," which is a parallel of the oath of Hippocrates but emphasizes more the spiritual importance of the statement. "As God is my witness, I dedicate my life to the welfare of my patients. No matter what the circumstances, I vow to do my best to provide appropriate counsel and proper medication to those who seek my services. With gratitude to God for the opportunity to serve humanity, I will make an effort to increase my knowledge and skills as I practice professional pharmacy. Putting aside all self-interests and pursuing righteousness at all times, I aspire to reflect God's mercy and compassion in caring for those suffering in body, mind, or spirit. I will respect the sanctity of life and will avoid any treatment that may deprive any human being of the gift of life. Always aware that God loves each of us and can foster healing of all diseases, I will encourage an attitude of hopefulness in all of my patients. I will remember that there is an art as well as a science to the practice of pharmacy and that warmth, sympathy, and understanding enhance the effectiveness of the medication I dispense" (published in *Christianity and Pharmacy*, volume 13, Fall/Winter 2010). Pharmacists as well as physicians feel it's a privilege to serve us who need their professional help.

A deep, abiding faith in God is key to all healing. Yet so many of us are trained to think logically or scientifically that we can't understand or trust anything else. Daniel Sulmasy is a man with a unique background who addresses this issue. He is a Franciscan friar as well as a physician

(Cornell, 1882). He completed his residency in general internal medicine at Johns Hopkins Hospital and in 1995 received a PhD in philosophy from Georgetown University. He comments that "the notion of miracles sits awkwardly inside the temple of scientific medicine." He adds that "skepticism about miracles is most common among scientifically educated persons." (D. Sulmasy, "What Is a Miracle?" *Southern Medical Journal* 1100: 1223, 2007). Sulmasy suggests that physicians should be taught to respect both science and the spirituality of the individual patient and to look for the best options to produce a positive clinical outcome. Ideally, it helps if the physician has some spiritual insight and can resonate with the patient on this basis. "Religion is the oldest form of medical practice." Between 33 and 77 percent of the people prefer to have a physician who is deeply spiritual and can relate to them on a spiritual basis (D. Sulmasy, "Spirituality, Religion and Clinical Care" *CHEST* 2009, 135:1634).

On the other hand, Dr. Sulmasy mentions that many medical schools already have included courses in spirituality and health care but this is a controversial area ("A Balm for Gilead," Georgetown University Press, Washington, DC, 2006). Some critics state that studies of the role of spirituality in health care are not good science. So we have a dilemma not only in the minds of most people but also among medical educators. Is disease a scientific or a spiritual problem?

Miracles are defined by Dr. Sulmasy as unusual real events, verifiable empirically, not magic and affirmed by people who believe in God. They are not violations of immutable physical laws. God not only created the universe but also sustains it from moment to moment, and he can alter those sustaining laws. Health-care students should be taught early on that miracles can and do occur especially under the right spiritual and evidence-based treatment conditions. One of the challenges of medical education and in medical practice in the USA today is to balance the rigid evidence-based approach with a more humane, faith-based approach. People need symmetric, levelheaded, holistic treatments to handle their health needs.

CHAPTER 2

Some Problems in Medicine Today

Excellence is the gradual result of always wanting to do better.
—Pat Riley

According to *Wikipedia*, life expectancy in the USA is 78.3 years, and we rank thirty-ninth compared to other countries. Japan is number one at 82.6 years. Also, health-care costs are by far greater in the USA than anywhere else. Yet the *NY Times* reported (August 12, 2007) that "many Americans are under the delusion that we have the best medical care in the world." Certainly our medical care is the most expensive in the world, but why do we not live as long as people in other countries?

Atul Gwande, a surgeon at Brigham and Woman's Hospital in Boston, stated that the "complexity of the field of medicine has developed to the point where it has exceeded the individual capacities of doctors." Addressing the 2009 graduating class at Harvard Medical School, he explained that doctors can no longer master the diagnosis of the tens of thousands of conditions that afflict human beings, the actions of six thousand drugs and the four hundred medical and surgical procedures available. Health personnel need to work together, and Dr. Gwande advocates a "pit crew" approach with checklists to ensure that all patients receive complete and appropriate care. Doctors have been "cowboys" to handle everything themselves, but what are needed now are pit crew people who will work together to eliminate the two million infections that occur annually in American hospitals and to cut in half the 188,000 deaths associated annually with surgery. Fellowship and teamwork are of critical importance.

Furthermore, behavioral and social sciences have been neglected in medical education for many years. We now realize that over half of all deaths in the United States are related to behavioral and social factors. Sedentary lifestyles and substance abuse are two of the main problems. "Biomedical research alone is not enough to unravel all the behavioral factors that contribute to these problems. Also, medical education often does not adequately address social and behavioral factors, missing the opportunity to reduce premature deaths and improve the quality of life for many" (Overview and Recommendations of the Behavioral and Social Science Work Group, IUSM Curriculum Committee, February 2012). The curriculum of the Indiana School of Medicine is being revised to include behavioral and social sciences to better serve the people of the state of Indiana. So plans for better education of American medical students in the social sciences area are already under way.

Lectures have been a main mechanism for teaching in universities for many years. However, lectures are thought to produce poor retention of didactic material and may be especially deficient in developing problem-solving skills. Alternatively, when small groups of students work together either in problem-based learning (PBL) or team-based learning (TBL), effectiveness of instruction is generally enhanced, and other skills like teamwork and interpersonal communication are improved. Our pharmacology course for medical students at Purdue is primarily a lecture-based approach. To enhance effectiveness of the course, we added four TBL open-book quizzes, covering new lecture material and offered a small amount of extra credit for good group performance. The students were not given a chance to study the material, but they took the quizzes individually and then retook them working in groups of about four. The quizzes were open-book so the students did not depend on memory to answer the questions but only used good judgment. We were hoping to promote interaction among students so they would learn from one another. Surprisingly, we found that there was variation in effectiveness of the groups. Some groups consistently improved on retaking the quizzes, and others consistently did not. These are all intelligent, well-rounded young people. The success of the group was not entirely related to academic ability since group performance was not correlated with how well the students in the group did in the pharmacology course as a whole. This illustrates the importance of good personal interactions among medical personnel. It's to the patient's advantage that physicians interact well with one another in making medical decisions.

Some of our medical students did not enjoy interacting with one another in the TBL quizzes. They preferred the old way of studying after the lectures and then taking the exams individually. The TBL quizzes, therefore, were important to get the students used to talking with one another about medical issues and to encourage them to become more like pit crew people and to care for us in the best way possible.

In many TBL exercises in medical schools, groups of ten to twelve are used because of large class sizes. Our group size may be more appropriate to some clinical practices since institutional physicians often consult with one another in groups of three to four regarding patient therapy, according to Cecelia May, hospitalist, St. Elizabeth's Heath Care, Lafayette, Indiana. In difficult cases, group size may be about five. So our groups of three to four are appropriate and relevant to some types of medical practice.

Ideally, all physicians should have a broad-based knowledge, the proper pit crew skills, and a lot of common sense. But this is not a perfect world. In the midst of a busy fall semester with all the pressure of lectures and a deeply emotional conflict with a friend at church, I had trouble breathing. I had to take shallow breaths because to breathe deeply was extremely painful. I went to the emergency room at a local hospital and was admitted with streptococcal pneumonia. The hospitalist explained that when the lungs become inflamed, it's painful when they rub against the rib cage on taking deep breaths. They gave me an antibiotic intravenously. I was in the hospital for four days.

My second night in the hospital, I was exhausted and desperately needed sleep. They gave me a roommate who stayed up all night long with the light on, working on his computer, making funny little noises. He explained he didn't want to go to sleep because he was afraid he would stop breathing if he fell asleep. Well, I couldn't sleep either. In the middle of the night, he ordered a dish of chocolate ice cream. I suggested to him that maybe if he repeated the name of Jesus over and over, he could sleep. He said, "Yah, maybe you're right," but he kept on working his computer. Also, the needle for the IV drip of the antibiotic came out of my blood vessel, my wrist began to swell, and the needle had to be reinserted. I slept very little that night and was even more tired than when I entered the hospital.

The next day I requested another room. Thank God there was one available, and I got a good night's sleep. One of the nurses commented that I looked a lot better than I did the day before. The bottom line is that there is a need for common sense in medical practice. Modern medical practice is very sophisticated, but shouldn't they have known that patients need a quiet room to get some sound, restful sleep? Thank God that many new hospitals have private rooms.

A good night's sleep is one of the best therapies. "Sleep disorders and sleep deficiency are important causes of adverse health effects and increased mortality in the United States and worldwide" (C. Czisler, J. Clin. *Sleep Med.* 2011, Oct 15;7 [5 Suppl]: S6-8). It's known that when rats are deprived of sleep, they don't live long. Normally they live two to three years, but without sleep, they live only five weeks. These sleep-deprived rats also develop sores on their skin. Apparently, tissue repair in skin and other organs occurs during normal restful sleep. Shouldn't a good night's sleep be a top priority of medical therapy and emphasized in medical treatment programs?

I have a close friend who had an unpleasant experience at the same hospital that treated me. She says the treatment she received did not reflect the Christian values this hospital claims to embrace. Her complaint is not against any individual but, rather, an attitude that ignores the rights of the patient to receive adequate information and does not respect the wishes of patients concerning their medical care. She describes her experience as follows:

On Friday, December 12, 2003, I began to feel quite fatigued and experienced a loss of appetite and nausea. I also had a cold (coughing, sneezing), so I thought I had the flu. There were a lot of news reports about the flu at this time, including some deaths. After experiencing no improvement, I called my doctor, on Monday, December 22, 2003, to schedule an appointment. I was told that she was busy that day and preparing to go on vacation, so I was assigned to see her nurse practitioner. During the office visit, I listed my three symptoms and she agreed that I had the flu. She told me to get plenty of rest and to drink plenty of liquids to prevent dehydration. Following the meeting, I went to work. Later in the afternoon, one of the chaplains sat down at my desk and said, "You look yellow," and abruptly got up and walked into her office. I thought she was kidding, so I didn't ask what she meant by yellow. I felt too ill to go to work the rest of the week.

On Sunday, December 28, 2003, I drove to my office to see how much work had piled up on my desk while I was absent. I was planning to return to work on Monday. After a few minutes, I walked over to the restroom and looked at myself in the mirror. I was surprised to see that I was quite jaundiced. Even the whites of my eyes were yellow. I had not seen anything like this before and did not know what it indicated. I was very scared. I went back to my office and talked to a priest, the chaplain who was working that day. I also decided to call the chaplain who had told me I looked yellow and ask if I should go to the ER. I was frightened since I had heard news reports that many people had died from the flu that I thought I had. It was the Sunday between Christmas and New Year. I didn't know what to do except go to the ER. The two chaplains agreed to accompany me there.

In the ER, the doctor asked me to describe my symptoms, so I told him about the extreme fatigue, loss of appetite, and nausea and that I had just noticed that I was jaundiced. He asked if I had been out of the country recently, and I told him that I had been in Mexico from November 16 to the twenty-second. I went with a church group to build houses for residents of a colonia in Mexico just across the Texas border. The doctor suggested I might have contracted hepatitis from eating contaminated food. He also mentioned in a nonchalant, matter-of-fact voice that I might have colon cancer. This was quite a shock since I thought I just had the flu.

One of the chaplains told the doctor that I did not have health insurance that year, but I was enrolled for 2004, just three and a half days away. The doctor responded that he does not recommend letting financial considerations affect his medical decisions. The doctor had some blood tests done and reported to me that I was anemic. He asked if I had experienced any abnormal rectal bleeding, and I responded that I had. (I have hemorrhoidal bleeding on occasion, but it lasts only a couple of days, so I had not been concerned about it). He suggested that I have an ultrasound performed. I really did not want this done. I really just wanted to leave and go home. I was experiencing no pain and didn't think I had something as horrible as cancer. I was reeling from the thought of having cancer and could not understand how the doctor could make a diagnosis with such a small amount of data and not knowing my medical history. However, with the doctor and the chaplains encouraging me, I reluctantly gave in to having the test.

When the ultrasound was finished, I was taken to the ER, and a short time later, the doctor came in. He told me it looked very serious and that he had discussed my case with a gastroenterologist. He suggested that I be admitted to the hospital and have a colonoscopy performed the next morning. I replied, "I want to go home." The doctor moved to within about four feet of my face, raised his voice in an angry tone, and said, "You can't go home. You could bleed to death tonight. You would never be able to make it to the phone in time to call 911." (One of the chaplains had told the doctor that I live alone.) I repeated "I want to go home." The doctor replied, still standing close to me and speaking in a raised voice, "I don't think you understand. You have one-third less blood than most people," and then pointed to the two chaplains who were with me in the room. I don't recall the exact words that were spoken after this. Given the choice between possibly bleeding to death and being admitted to the hospital to have a colonoscopy the very next morning, I reluctantly agreed to be admitted to the hospital.

Later, in August 2004 I talked with a person in human relations at the hospital about my experience in the ER. When I expressed my concern that the doctor had focused on colon cancer instead of the more likely hepatitis, she said that "doctors always look for the worst-case scenario in order to avoid possible lawsuits." It seems to me, if that is indeed what the doctor did, then he ignored his own advice and made a decision based on financial considerations. I believe this is unjust and unchristian.

As I was taken to the hospital room, I was determined to tell the nurse or whoever I was to meet there that I really didn't want to be admitted to the hospital and undergo the colonoscopy. I was hoping to find someone who would listen to me and discuss my concerns. So when the nurse came into the room, I told her that I wanted to go home. She snapped back, "You can't do that." I did not respond. She said nothing further.

Once again, I had encountered a medical professional who ignored me, who did not take the time to talk to me and learn what I wanted to do regarding my medical care. Also, I was horribly weak, fatigued, and nauseated after drinking a gallon of liquid to prepare for the test. It was inhumane treatment. My body did not need that distress and discomfort.

In the morning of December 29, I was taken to have the colonoscopy. I expected to have time to talk with the doctor who was to perform the procedure, and I was hoping that I could convince him not to do the exam now but allow me to wait until the results of the hepatitis test were known. The doctor, however, did not want to discuss it and ignored my comments. So the colonoscopy was performed and negative results were obtained. The next day, the results of the hepatitis test came back positive. I was released from the hospital on the thirty-first still feeling weak but relieved that I did not have colon cancer.

Unfortunately, a few weeks later, the bill for the unnecessary ultrasound and colonoscopy and the hospital stay arrived. It amounted to $15,000, approximately 100 percent of my yearly salary as receptionist in pastoral care at the hospital. If only the doctors could have postponed the tests a couple of days and allowed me to go home and rest, that expense could have been avoided. Also, the health benefits of going home to rest would have been great. All this occurred in a Christian hospital whose employees are "encouraged to do their best to care for their patients and their families, to treat them in a way they would want their loved ones to be treated."

So despite all our sophisticated powerful drugs, fancy diagnostic procedures, modern treatments, and good intentions, there is a great need for more common sense and good TBL-type human interaction in the medical care program. We should address these needs early on in the medical education process.

You've probably heard the little jingle grade-school kids sing, "The six best doctors anywhere and no one can deny it are sunshine, water, rest and air and exercise and diet." Presumably, when they mention *rest*, that also includes sleep. Despite the wisdom in this little jingle, obesity in our country is rampant, people watch too much TV, are addicted to alcohol, tobacco or drugs, and we all worry too much because of so little faith in a loving, compassionate God. We've forgotten these simple lessons of Sunday school and do what we think is right often ignoring sunshine, water, rest and air and exercise and diet. Medical education in this country of ours may be adequate overall with some improvements needed, but also, Americans appear to lack spiritual strength.

CHAPTER 3

What on Earth Are You Doing, for God's Sake?

Unless the Lord build the house, they labor in vain that build it.
—Psalm 127:1

How did I get where I am? As I look back from the vantage point of seventy-nine years, I'm amazed at what I'm doing. I can't believe I'm teaching medical students. I'm a shy person, not very outgoing. When I went to high school, I didn't say anything in class for two years. I had always been the quiet one who just listens to what others have to say. How could I possibly earn a PhD and lecture to medical students? Could I please digress and explain how I miraculously got into the position I now have by mentioning my family background, schooling, and early work experience?

My dad was born in Eastern Germany in 1906. He told us that he remembered hearing the artillery firing when he went to bed at night as a child. He lived in a refugee camp for a while and remembers playing soccer there with the other kids. With the war, schooling was disrupted, so my dad had little education. There was a famine in Germany after the war, so many people migrated to the USA. Dad came to the USA at the age of seventeen with his brother Felix, who was nineteen. They settled in Columbus, Ohio, where their older brother, Leo, had preceded them and owned/operated a slaughterhouse. My dad actually worked for Uncle Leo, but money was scarce during the Great Depression, and sometimes, Dad would receive no pay. One of the other workers in the slaughterhouse was Fredrick Grundei, who had a daughter Anna Louise, who became my mother. So we were always poor since Dad only worked as a manual laborer. He was a reliable man though, a good husband and father.

Attending Catholic grade school and high school provided a firm religious background. Somehow, however, the real power and significance of Christianity passed me by. The bus ride of an hour to and from my all-boys high school was tedious. Also, I was the youngest and one of the smallest in the class and was embarrassed by living in a poor neighborhood. Once, when I was a senior, the guys offered me a ride home in their car. I tried to refuse, but they insisted. When we got to my house, they said, "Is this where you live?" It was embarrassing. The other boys had lawyers and physicians and dentists for fathers, and my dad worked as a coach cleaner on the Pennsylvania Railroad. Bullies in the neighborhood and some at school were a problem. It was not fun. But still, I'm grateful for the fine education I did have. I struggled to keep up with my schoolwork but graduated in the upper third of my class in high school.

A college education was cheap in those days, only $40 a quarter, and I paid for it myself by working second trick (3:00 to 11:00 p.m.) on the railroad. An aptitude test at Ohio State indicated that I was suited for science, so I enrolled in pharmacy. I lived at home and paid my parents $25 a month in room and board. I was fascinated with pharmacology and obtained the only A in a class of twenty-three students in one course. I thought I had some natural talent for pharmacology. Also, the guinea pig ileum lab was amazing to me, showing that a piece of gut could respond to drugs in a muscle bath with proper physiological salts, just as it does in the body. I knew I wanted to be a pharmacologist. The graduate students and postdoctoral fellows at Ohio State told me that it was better to get the PhD in a medical school rather than in a pharmacy school. However, Purdue Pharmacy School had a good graduate pharmacology program, so they suggested that I get a master's degree there first.

The master's degree was completed by the end of 1956. Dean Jenkins at Purdue, a fine, strong man who established the pharmacy school as a first-class research institution, was not happy when I said I wanted to get my PhD in a medical school. In my naïveté, I didn't realize I was insulting the man. Anyway, with great trepidation, I drove from West Lafayette, Indiana, to Chicago that winter to enter the Department of Pharmacology at Northwestern University Medical School. Dr. C. Jeleff Carr, pharmacology chairman at Purdue, recommended me to Dr. Carl Dragstedt, chairman at Northwestern. Both these men were really outstanding pharmacologists. Dr. Carr had written a pharmacology textbook, and Dr. Dragstedt was world renowned in the area of histamine pharmacology.

So I left a "college in a cornfield" atmosphere and came to the big city. The medical school is just a few blocks from Rush Street in Chicago with all its saloons and nightclubs. There was only one vacancy in the entire eight-story dormitory residence, Abbott Hall on Lake Shore Drive, and I had to share a room with a dental student who really didn't want me there. He had had the room to himself before I came. Competing with medical students was not easy. They study all the time. But I thought I could handle it. I even presented my master's work at the federation meetings there in Chicago that spring. However, I did poorly on the physiology quiz that following Monday. (We had a quiz every Monday.) I got a 67 percent. I barely made the required 80 percent average to get a B in the course. (The med students could get a C in the course and still pass.) By the grace of God, I made it through.

To obtain industrial experience, the faculty at Northwestern suggested that I spend the summer at Abbott Labs in North Chicago, Illinois, in the Pharmacology Division, headed by Dr. Richard K. Richards, an MD from Germany. He had a program there for drug development, and anticonvulsants were being emphasized at that time. A group of chemists synthesized new compounds, and a variety of animals including primates was used to evaluate the effects of these agents. They helped develop trimethadione and valproate, still available today for petit mal epilepsy. They had me injecting mice with a monoamine oxidase inhibitor and then giving amphetamine or DOPA (dihydroxy phenylalanine, used for treatment of parkinsonism) to cause a wild, manic stimulation of the mice. They would actually kill each other after this treatment. Drugs have powerful effects on the brain. I felt very insecure, however, since I needed a PhD research project, and I had no idea what to do. Also, my faith in God was weak, and I had no real spiritual foundation.

As a very naive young man with so many adjustments to make in a short time, it was difficult. I stayed in the YMCA in North Chicago. I started dating a girl who was Dr. Richards's secretary. She was two and a half years older than I. Being extremely insecure, I became emotionally attached to her very rapidly. She lived in a house with some other young ladies and represented maturity and stability to me. We went to outdoor summer concerts and went to the beach and to movies. She even took me to her home and introduced me to her mother. It was fun. But she could see I really didn't have things together and informed me that she just didn't think our relationship would work. I was devastated. With the rejection and all the pressure of graduate school, it was just too much for me. I couldn't sleep or eat well, and I couldn't function well. At a time when I needed God the most, I made a foolish decision, I stopped going to church. I blamed God for all that happened. It's a wonder I made it through the PhD program. I'm so grateful to Dr. Dragstedt and to my adviser, Dr. William C. North, for their understanding. It took years to sort out all the emotional trauma.

To make a long story short, I left Northwestern to serve six months of active duty as an officer in the United States Army Reserve in San Antonio, Texas, and afterward was employed as a toxicologist at Brooks Air Force base in Texas. Then I did postdoctoral work at Harvard Medical School under Norman Weiner, MD, a very intelligent man and a fine researcher. I also taught pharmacology for five years at the medical school associated with Wake Forest University in Winston Salem, North Carolina, and then came back to Purdue. I owe Dr. Tom Miya and Dean Varro Tyler much appreciation for hiring me. They were very generous and welcoming. Purdue is a fine university. Only on returning to Purdue did I resume church attendance and begin to sort out all my emotional refuse. The Charismatic Christian movement came to the Purdue campus the same time I did in 1969. I don't think this was a coincidence, but it was God's way of calling me home.

Please let me mention a significant event that occurred in the state of Indiana in the 1960s. Indiana ranked in the lower third of the United

States in number of physicians per one hundred thousand population at that time. In 1965, the state legislature arrived at a consensus to build a second medical school. The cost was estimated at $150 million. However, every section of Indiana wanted the school in their area, and also, the money was not available. So a commission was created to devise a plan that would solve the problem. Among the members of the commission was Beurt SerVaas, president of the Indianapolis City Council. He had a degree in chemistry from Indiana University (IU) and was licensed to teach in high school in Indiana. Also, he was working on a PhD in medical science from IU School of Medicine. After several meetings and public hearings, the commission could come to no agreement. SerVaas proposed that small medical centers be created around the state at already existing universities. This would greatly reduce building costs and provide instruction from resident faculty. The idea was rejected by the commission but was included in the appendix of the report.

The plan was submitted to the newly elected governor of Indiana, Ed Whitcomb. He was inclined to sign the Medical Education Authority Bill since it had approval from the legislature. However, he began to receive phone calls from all over the state objecting to the plan. He also had his own reservations especially regarding the enormous cost, which would bankrupt the state of Indiana. The governor noticed the item in the appendix and thought it was the best solution. So he appointed Beurt SerVaas as chairman of a State Medical Education Commission.

However, the needs were urgent (fourteen months' time), and there was no budget. SerVaas accepted the job anyway and said he could do it by using his own finances. He accomplished the goal! It was a miracle and provided an immediate increase in medical class size at a minimum of cost. It seems God had a plan, and things happened quickly and efficiently for the benefit of the people of the state of Indiana. The timing of the establishment of the regional Indiana medical programs also fit perfectly with my appearance on the Purdue campus.

Why all this background? Only to say that my experiences, illogical and traumatic though they were, all fit well with my present position at Purdue. It was necessary that I get a PhD at a medical school because one of my main jobs here at Purdue has been teaching medical students. I needed to have my heart broken by that young lady in North Chicago. Otherwise, I never would have understood the great importance of love in my life. Also I never would have understood the meaning of the first commandment. I would have put that lady ahead of God. I would have worshiped her and not the God of the universe. This man/woman idea was an important part of God's plan, and he uses it for his own purposes. When I left the Catholic Church, I attended services of many other denominations. I needed to develop an appreciation for each part of the ecumenical church. Had I remained a Catholic all my life, I would not have been able to relate well with other Christian faculty and students here at Purdue. Also, the Charismatic movement, with all its emphasis on divine physical healing, gave me insight into the role of spirituality in the healing process. Physical healings were an important part of Jesus's ministry, and he took a positive attitude toward all those who came to him in their need.

As it says in the catechism of the Catholic Church, we're here on this planet earth to get to know, love, and serve God. Our lives are not a series of random events but have a serious purpose. Even when we don't recognize it or appreciate it, we are guided so we can be of greatest value to God here on earth. Everyone is important, and we should all work together for our mutual benefit. As I look back on my life, I can see where my experiences have prepared me for what I do now. These events were guideposts conducting me along a narrow path so that I can now serve my fellow man in a way, hopefully, pleasing to God. Even my mistakes, failures, and sins have provided important lessons.

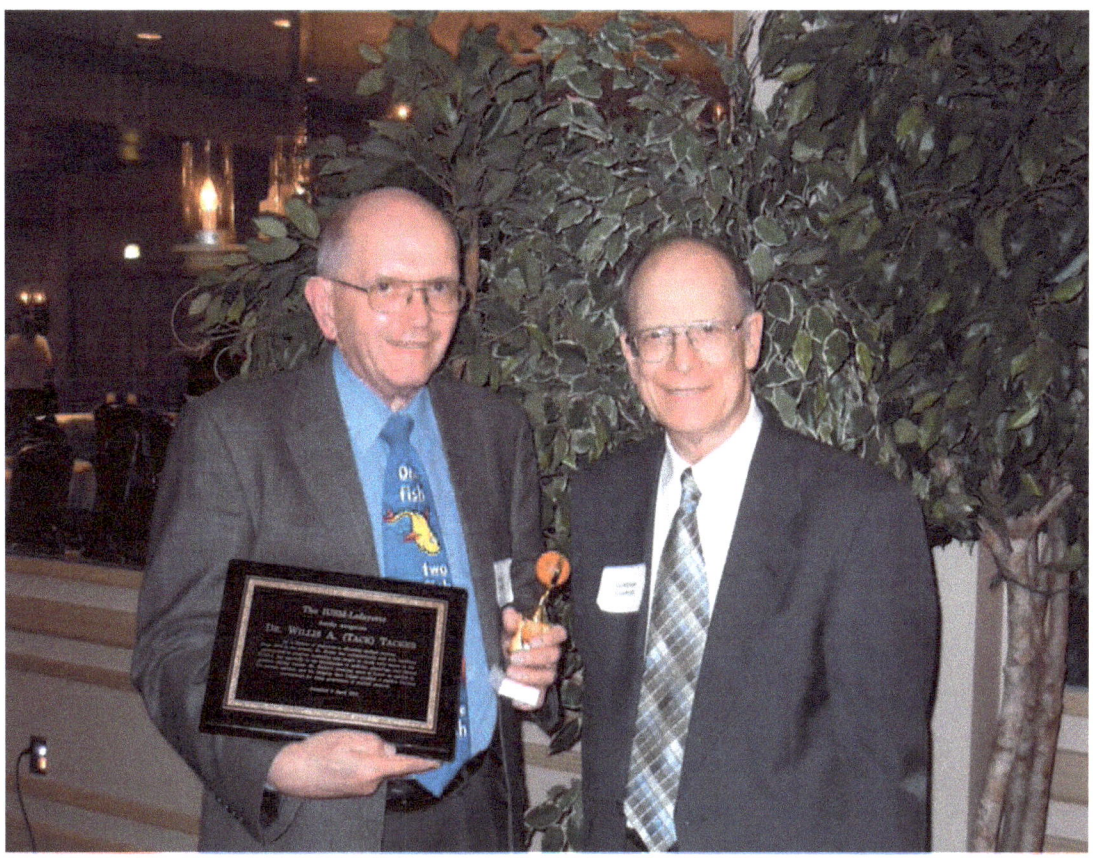

On the right is our present Dean Gordon Coppoc DVM, PhD at the 2011 Spring Dinner for our Lafayette Center medical program. He has been Dean for about 16 years and does a fine job. He is shown presenting an Award to Dr. Willis Tacker MD, PhD for his contributions to our program. Dr. Tacker gave a deeply moving presentation at the Spring Dinner on the occasion of his retirement. He quoted Shakespeare telling the students that you are the "stuff of my dreams". He devoted his life to educating these brilliant young people to enable them to help people with health problems.

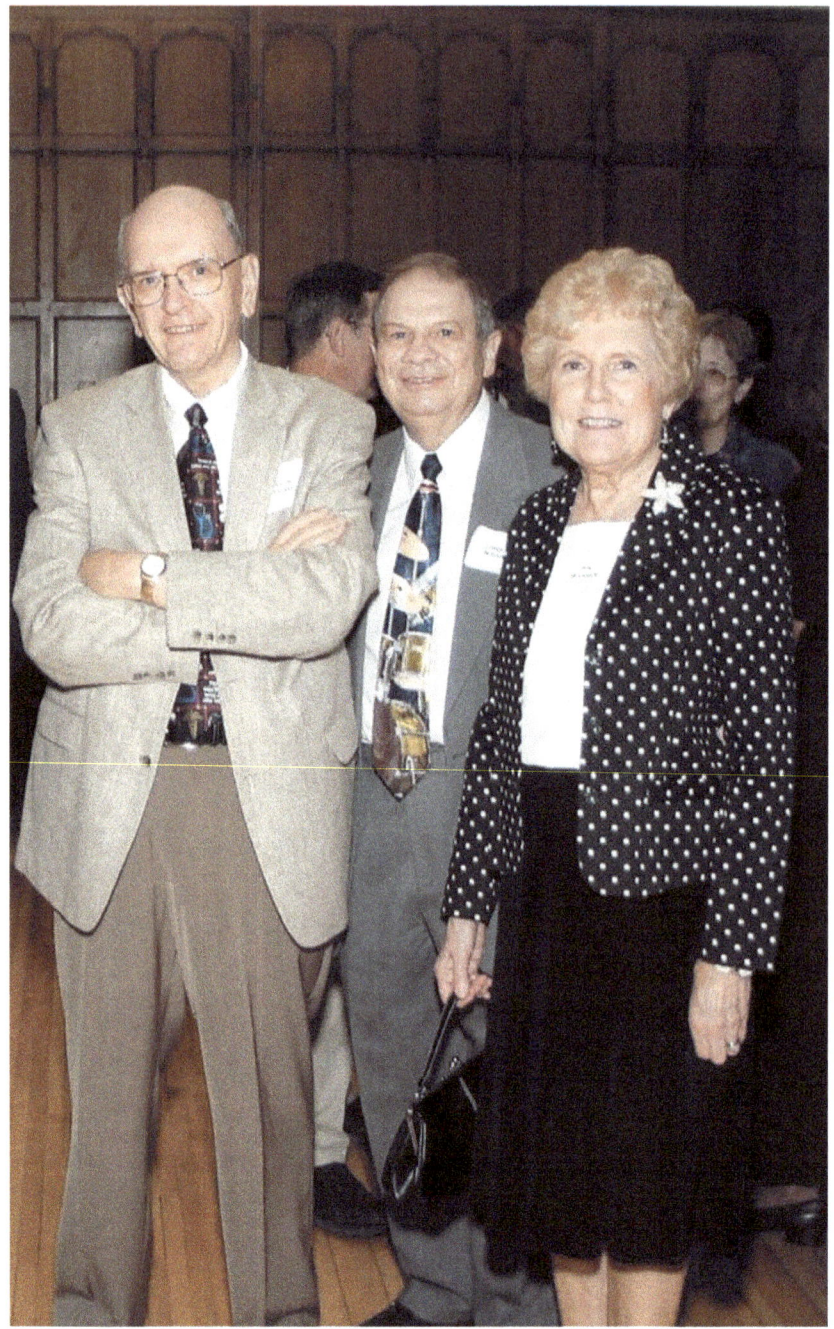

Willis Tacker MD, PhD Professor of Medicine at our Lafayette Center not only a fine person but also a great teacher and a good clinician. With him are Lindley Wagner MD and Mrs Wagner. Dr. Wagner was our first Dean at the Lafayette Center and got us started on the right foot and provided a good foundation for us to grow on.

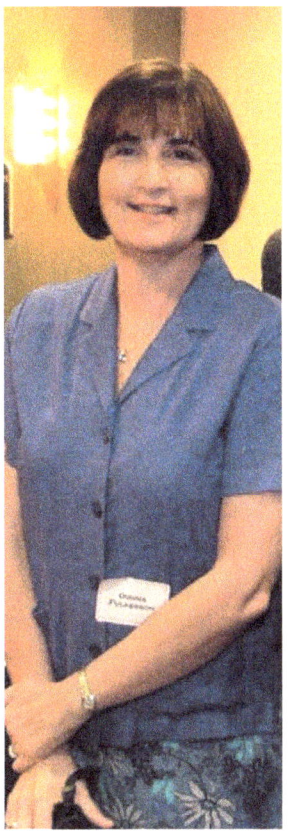

Donna Fulkerson was Head Secretary for Dean Coppoc for many years. She has been very helpful to the medical students and also to the faculty. We all appreciated her efficient presence in our program.

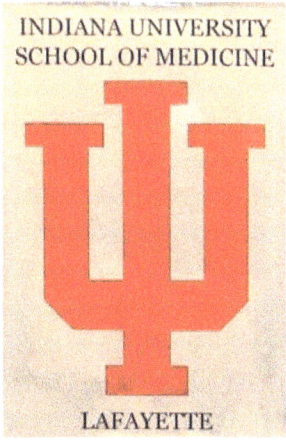

This is the official Logo for our Lafayette Center for Medical Education.

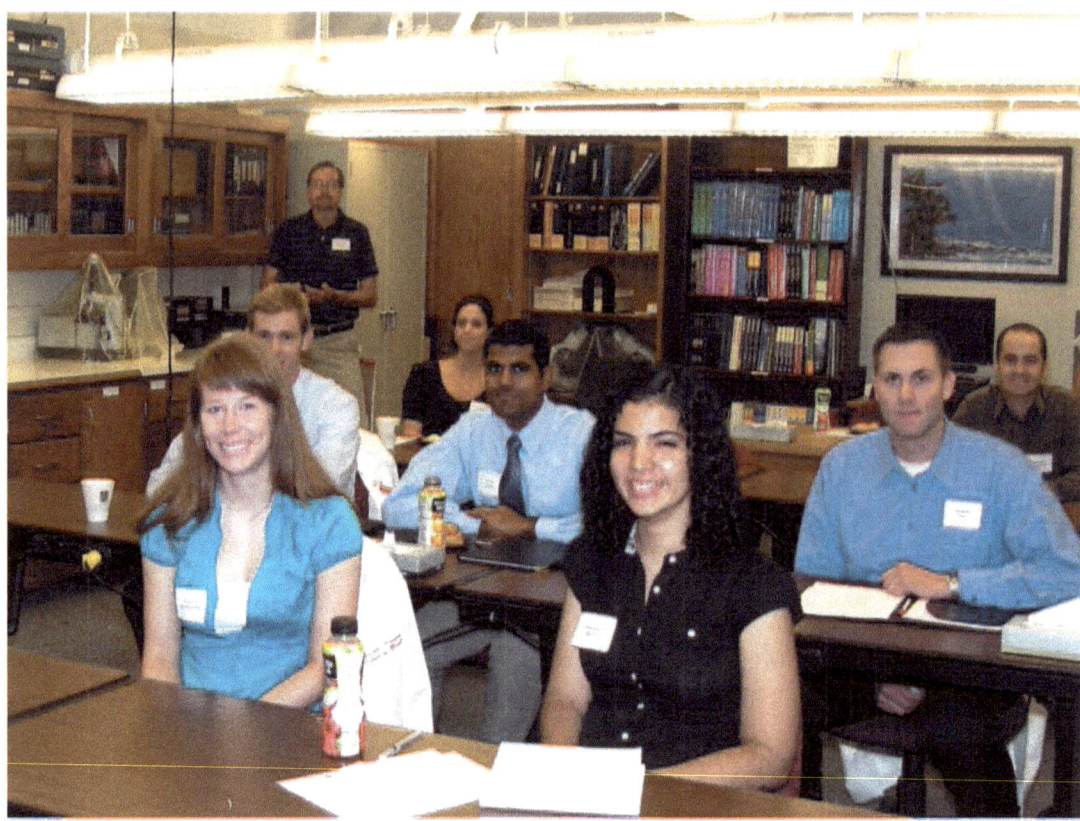

Classroom Scene Lafayette Center for Medical Education This is a view of about half of one of the classrooms at our small medical center. We see several students from left to right, Sarah Badenhop, Chris Bodle, Hari Vasu, Jarrod Day, and Brenton Goodman. Faculty member standing in the back is John Turek. The person next to Dr. Turek is Dr. Tacker's daughter Katherine, an MD from the University of Washington. The classrooms were very comfortable for the students and very workable for the faculty.

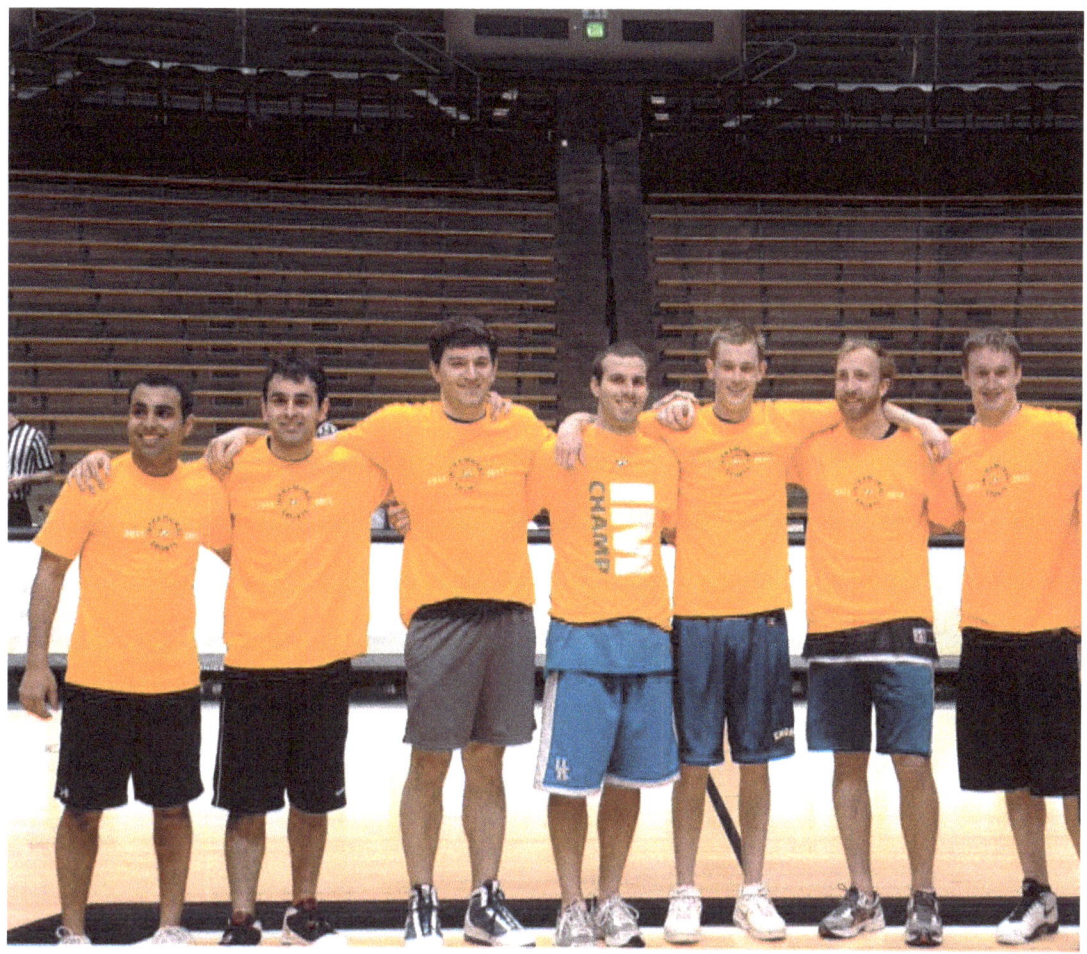

Purdue Intramural Basketball Championship 2012. Our medical students formed a team and signed up for Intramural Basketball at Purdue competing with top notch graduate and undergraduate students. They did well and entered the Intramural Championship Match. They won easily with Drew Schmidt sinking many three-pointers. He was selected "Most Valuable Player". The others did well too with Cody Bearden gathering in many rebounds. Pictured from left to right are Zahab Ahsan, Murad Arif, Jordan Marz, Drew Schmidt, Chris Bodle, Paul Wilson, and Cody Bearden.

CHAPTER 4

The Proper Motivation Is Essential

After the madness of the cross, any other madness is timid indeed.
—Jacques Maritain

Some golf professionals were talking about President Obama and thought that he was too busy with important things to play golf. One pro commented that he thought it was OK for Obama to play golf. He said Obama should suffer just like the rest of us. Golf is hard and so is life. We need all the help we can get. When you're young, you think you can do anything; you're smart, strong, and are going to live forever. You've got the world by a string. If we're wise though, we know not to trust ourselves. We need to appreciate authority, to see the big picture, and understand that people need to fit in and be a part of a team in order to be effective in this world. Some people, including myself, take years to come to this realization. Please let me explain.

At the age of forty-two, I was an associate professor at Purdue University. I had a fine, interesting job teaching and doing research. I did not attend church regularly although I was raised in the Catholic faith. Mostly, I was just like other people doing what I could to get ahead with a "me first" attitude. I was married to a fine lady and had two outstanding young sons, yet I was not really happy. One Friday, another associate professor, Dr. Don Blake, who had the office across mine, suggested that I go to a Full Gospel Business Men's meeting on that weekend (second week in October 1978). I knew Dr. Blake was happy deep down, but I thought he was a little strange with a Bible on his desk and always talking about Jesus. We played handball together, and afterward, he was talking about Christianity. I was embarrassed since the locker room was crowded. This reflects where I was spiritually. I didn't want to go to the Full Gospel meeting, but my family was out of town, and I had nothing else to do.

The speaker was a former state policeman from Georgia. He was doing well in his job and had a nice family with two little daughters. His mother was worried about him though since he did not go to church. One day, his wife asked him to say the blessing before the meal. He said he didn't think he had to thank God for the meal since he himself had earned the money to pay for it. His wife was disappointed with him, and as you might expect, this man was headed for trouble. He began having problems with alcohol and sometimes went to work with alcohol on his breath. Not a good thing for a state policeman who patrols the highways and is often one of the first at the scene of an accident.

This man went home from work one day and found a note from his wife saying she had taken the two daughters and left him. She couldn't stand it any longer. He was terribly hurt since he loved his wife very much. He felt deeply rejected and angry. Not having God for consolation, he took matters in his own hands and, with his police .38-caliber pistol, went looking for his family. He was so upset and felt so betrayed; he was going to shoot his wife and two little daughters; those two little girls that

God had given him. Fortunately, he couldn't find them. So dejected and discouraged was he that he drove his car out on a lonely country road in Georgia, and he put that gun barrel in his mouth and pulled the trigger. The gun misfired. In his hurt and abandonment, he again put that gun barrel in his mouth and again pulled the trigger. Another misfire. He was amazed because that weapon was well maintained and reliable. He rolled down the car window and fired the gun out the window. It worked fine. He knew something miraculous had happened and that his mother was praying for him. There on that lonely country road in Georgia, he broke down and wept for some time and felt the presence of the Holy Spirit. This experience changed his life, and he knew God was calling him to a life of service.

He was able to overcome his addiction to alcohol, and his job performance as a policeman improved. In fact, he was selected as one of those assigned to protect the governor of Georgia. At that time, that was Jimmy Carter, who later became president of the United States. How God puts his people in influential positions. This man was able to encourage Jimmy Carter in his Christian faith.

After giving up alcohol, this man was reunited with his family. One of his daughters went down to a neighbor lady and told her that she had a new daddy. She knew that this man was not the same as before. Children are especially sensitive to what is deep within people's hearts. When the Holy Spirit comes into your whole being, you become a new person, old things are passed away and all things are made new. This man resigned from the state police force, went to Bible college, and became a preacher of the Gospel. There wasn't a dry eye in the room that second Saturday in October 1978 when the speaker invited people to come forward for baptism in the Holy Spirit. I'm a shy person, but I knew I needed that baptism, and I actually ran up to the front despite the crowd of people. It was a life-changing experience. I finally found some peace, and the Holy Scriptures took on greater meaning. I started attending prayer meetings and teaching Sunday school and being more active in the Catholic Church. This experience also had a great effect on my professional life and influenced my approach to teaching pharmacology to medical and pharmacy students. Therefore, this was an important story to share with you at the beginning of this book and leads me into a description of the Charismatic movement, which is so important in my personal and professional life.

Full Gospel Business Men's Fellowship International (FGBFI) is a Pentecostal organization that believes in the power of the Holy Spirit to heal and guide and comfort those who deeply believe. They think what the Bible says is true. That's why they are called Full Gospel. There's no holding back, and everyone who believes in the resurrected Christ is welcome. Housewives are considered businessmen and are also welcome as members.

FGBFI is part of the Charismatic movement. According to the Internet, "The Charismatic movement is an international Christian renewal program and one of the most popular and fastest growing forces in the Christian world today." The movement traces its roots to the Azusa Street Mission in Los Angeles, California, at a Methodist-sponsored revival in the early 1900s. From there, the movement slowly spread throughout the whole world, and many were baptized in the Holy Spirit and experienced joy and healing. After the death of its founder, Demos Shakarian, in 1993, FGBFI has fragmented and is not so well coordinated today.

Unfortunately, the Charismatic movement has also diminished in the USA over the last thirty-five years due in part to the failure of some renowned TV evangelists. Oral Roberts, Jimmy Swaggart, John Bertoluchi, and Jim Bakker were powerful, charismatic, effective men of God but were enticed by their own desires and were led astray. Much as young King Solomon was a godly, righteous man but was led astray by the Canaanite religion as he grew older and more successful. Men make mistakes. This does not disprove the power of the Holy Spirit. I know several Spirit-filled people who are righteous, respectable citizens and a credit to their communities. Ministers filled with the Holy Spirit are able to inspire and bring joy to their congregations. On the other hand, I know some pastors who do not believe in divine healing and who apparently are not Spirit-filled and are very ineffective. One, in particular, comes to mind, who was pedantic, gave bland, pompous sermons, and sweated profusely in the process.

All three synoptic Gospels have the story of the calming of the sea. Matthew 8:26 says that suddenly a great tempest arose on the sea so that the boat was covered with waves. But Jesus was asleep. Then his disciples woke him, saying, "Lord save us! We are perishing." But he said to them, "Why are you fearful, O you of little faith?" Then he arose and rebuked the winds and the sea, and there was a great calm. The men marveled at him, saying, "Who can this be that the winds and the seas obey him?" What Jesus was really saying was that you guys need to get beyond yourselves; you need to think of the big picture. You're here for a great purpose, the salvation of mankind. In fact, most of you are going to sacrifice your lives, but don't worry about that; think of the magnificent project you are involved in. They couldn't face up to the task until they had received the Holy Spirit on Pentecost. We also need the Holy Spirit to face up to the challenges before us. He is the power and the courage and the wisdom of God enabling us to overcome all the obstacles before us and to avoid being overly concerned with ourselves.

Without a firm spiritual basis, it is not possible for ministers, doctors, teachers, or anyone else to live joyful, productive lives. This is a great privilege, and many people have given their very lives for the right to lead deeply spiritual lives. Franz Jagerstatter, who died for his faith at the hands of the Nazis in World War II, said, "I can say from my own experience how painful life often is when one lives as a halfway Christian; it is more like vegetating than living." Louis Lallemant said that a man of prayer will accomplish more in a year's apostolate than another in a lifetime. Also Billy Graham says, "A life without God is like an unsharpened pencil, it has no point to it." A godly motivation is critical for success, happiness, and contentment in any occupation here on earth.

CHAPTER 5

Divine Healing

Jesus went about all the cities and villages, teaching in their synagogues, preaching the gospel of the kingdom, and healing every sickness and every disease among the people.

—Matthew 9:35

Not only do I teach medical students, but I also am faculty adviser to the Purdue Pharmacy Christian Student Association (PPCSA). I try to facilitate our weekly Bible study/prayer group to emphasize concepts applicable to pharmacy practice. It's a critical time for these young pharmacists. They are overwhelmed with all the science and technology in their seven-year program. They tend to forget the human aspect of the profession. We remind them that pharmacists deal primarily with broken, hurting people who are in need of compassion and sympathy and struggle with their faith and lack of hope. A positive attitude and belief in divine healing are critical for both doctors and pharmacists.

Each semester, we have speakers come to share with PPCSA. A pivotal talk was given by John Turek, associate dean of the Purdue School of Veterinary Medicine. He shared his missionary experience in a small village in India. The people there are Hindus who believe in many gods. Dr. Turek told them that there is only one God, and the one true God is powerful. The people believed Dr. Turek, and when he prayed for them, the blind were made to see and the deaf to hear and the lame to walk just as in the time of Christ. It was an amazing thing for Dr. Turek to witness. He is a good Christian and a man of great faith, but still, he was astonished at the healings that occurred when these people deeply believed. There is a great need for individuals in our time to deepen their faith and adopt a positive, hopeful, godly attitude. Medical professionals should encourage an optimistic outlook and deep belief in the power of the Holy Spirit to heal.

Our PPCSA president that year was a bright young man, Cory Smith, who went through the leadership program at Purdue. No one else wanted to be president, and he apparently thought it would look good on his resumé. So he volunteered. He wasn't very spiritual, but the meetings went OK anyway, just as some churches function well even if the church leadership is not especially spiritual. However, when this man heard the testimony of Dr. Turek, he was deeply affected and eventually became a firm believer. God has his ways of drawing us all close to himself.

Rev. Norman Vincent Peale, the famous evangelist, has shed insight onto the importance of prayer in the healing process. He tells of being awakened by the telephone at 3:00 a.m. It was a physician friend of his who was at the bedside of a patient from Dr. Peale's congregation. She was in a coma, and her doctor, a competent physician, had done everything medically he could for her. Still, she was not responding. He asked Dr. Peale to come over to the woman's house to help. Dr. Peale went to the lady's bedside and positioned himself on one side with the physician on the other. They alternately recited healing scripture passages, often quoting verses verbatim they had not memorized. They realized that patients can hear even if they are in a coma. This went on until the morning sun arose. Then, the patient stirred and opened her eyes and went to sleep. The physician said she had come out of the coma and was sleeping normally. He thanked Dr. Peale for his help in bringing about a miracle in this patient. There is a close connection between body and mind, and the proper mental attitude is important for healing to take place. Scripture passages have a powerful effect on our mental state.

Divine healing is important and obviously can occur without the aid of a physician or a pharmacist. A famous healing evangelist, Smith Wigglesworth, was born in England in 1859. Even as a boy, he was a godly person but was uneducated and started working as a plumber with his father at the age of seven. Child labor was common in those days. In 1889, he married Polly Featherstone, a vivacious young woman with a gift for preaching and evangelism. She taught him to read and write. They opened a mission where she preached, and he prayed for people to be healed. In 1907, this uneducated man was baptized in the Holy Spirit at the age of forty-eight and manifested new power to preach and began a worldwide healing ministry. He conducted healing services in the USA, Australia, South Africa, and all over Europe up to the time of his death in 1947.

This simple, uneducated man had a deep compassion for the sick and great faith that God could heal any and all illnesses by the power of the Holy Spirit. He was steadfast and firm in his beliefs. To give an example, some of Smith Wigglesworth's friends in London called him to minister to a twenty-six-year-old man who had been bedridden for eighteen years. He could not dress himself. Because of his inactivity, his legs were thin and his body enlarged. His parents had gotten him out of bed and dressed him when Smith came. He looked at the boy, and the situation seemed hopeless. He prayed for guidance from above and commanded the young man to rise up and walk. Nothing happened. Then the father and Smith tried to lift the boy to see if his legs would support him, but they could not move him. Then Smith again prayed for guidance and again commanded him to rise and walk by the power of the Holy Spirit. But no, he never walked. He rose and ran! He ran out the front door across the road and into a field and ran up and down and came back. The whole family was astounded and grateful. This may be interpreted as a psychosomatic phenomenon, but many other hard-core physical ailments were also healed through Smith Wigglesworth's intercessory prayer.

Another instance of healing involved a lady in Switzerland who had a goiter, an obviously enlarged thyroid. She was prayed for and then publicly thanked God for the healing. She came back to the healing service again the next year and thanked God for the healing. She did the same the following year although no change had occurred in the size of the goiter. The people asked her, "Haven't you looked in a mirror? Your goiter is as big as ever." She went home and prayed to the Lord. She said she knew she was healed, but the people doubted since there was no change in the size of the goiter, and she asked the Lord to help. The next morning, the goiter had shrunk, and she appeared normal. One more time she went to Smith Wigglesworth's meeting and thanked God for the healing. There is an important lesson here. The healing doesn't depend on appearances; it comes from deep within the soul. God in his time makes all things whole.

As he was leaving a healing meeting in Switzerland, two boys mentioned to Smith Wigglesworth that a blind man was at the meeting that day, but no one prayed for him. The blind man had heard all the words at the meeting and believed he would be healed that day and would not leave until he could see. Smith went to him and was told he had been blind from birth. Being pleased with his determination, Smith anointed him and touched his eyes, and for the first time in his life, this man was able to see. At first, he saw the electric lights in the room, and he counted them. Then he counted the people around him. The man was ecstatic. He looked at his watch to tell the time. For years, he had been touching the dials to determine the time. Realizing he had never seen the faces of his mother or father, he rushed out looking like someone awakened from a long, strange sleep. I'm sure Smith Wigglesworth was impressed by what happened, and can you imagine the joy of all the people who knew the man healed of blindness?

It is of utmost importance that physicians and pharmacists learn to appreciate the phenomenon of divine healing even in their early years of training. It is also important that patients themselves understand divine healing since they have primary responsibility for their own health. Physicians and pharmacists cannot bear the burden of all the ailments of their patients. They are expert advisers and well-meaning friends. They are duty bound to help in every way they can, but the main responsibility is on the patients themselves. Even the great Buddha made the statement that every human being is the author of their own health and disease. A genuine, positive hope and faith are needed by patients, their families, friends, and by all health professionals in attendance. Medical personnel need to encourage the proper attitude in their patients. We must all never forget that the risen Christ is with each one of us and he loves us, wants the best for all of us, and will never abandon us.

People can be ungrateful. Remember, when Christ healed the ten lepers, only one returned to thank him. Physicians and pharmacists are aware of this and need to keep the following in mind.

People are unreasonable, illogical, and self-centered.

    Love them anyway.

If you do good, people will accuse you of selfish ulterior motives.

    Do good anyway.

If you are successful, you will win false friends and true enemies.

    Succeed anyway.

Honesty and frankness make you vulnerable.

    Be honest and frank anyway.

The good you do will be forgotten tomorrow.

    Do good anyway.

People with the biggest ideas can be shot down by people with small minds.

    Think big anyway.

What you spend years building might be destroyed overnight.

    Build anyway,

Give the world the best you have and you'll get kicked in the teeth.

    Give the world the best you've got anyway.

CHAPTER 6

Spiritual Warfare

Rejoice in hope, be patient in tribulation, and continue steadfastly in prayer.

—Romans 12:12

A book on spirituality and health would not be complete without mention of spiritual warfare. Everyone knows about angels and demons, but many people in the USA don't believe they exist. They are "blinded by materialism and believe only in what they can see, hear, taste, smell, or touch." Theologian and biblical scholar Walter Wink, however, expands on the idea that spirits exist and says that "every business, corporation, school, denomination, bureaucracy, sports team, etc., is a combination of both the physical and the spiritual." In his book *The Powers That Be* (Doubleday, New York, 1998), he says that all human organizations have spirits associated with them. "There is nothing from DNA to the United Nations that does not have God as its core." Some spirits are beneficial; others are not.

Governments that are oppressive have evil spirits (Chile in 1982, South Africa in 1985, India in 1940) and use violence to maintain themselves.

When peaceful, nonviolent means are employed, these oppressive spirits can be combated and miracles can occur; the Berlin Wall comes down, South Africa and India were liberated, and equal rights are established in the southern United States.

For centuries, oppressive powers have been sustained by violence, which Wink refers to as the "domination system, sustained by the myth that violence is redemptive." Wink argues that Jesus's gospel is God's answer to the domination system. "Jesus himself broke the endless spiral of violence by absorbing its impact in his own flesh," a beautiful demonstration of the proper way to handle oppression. It shows the power of the living God in the resurrection and explains the persistence of the Christian faith for over two thousand years. Ultimately, God is in control.

The Bible warns us to "take on the whole armor of God that you may be able to stand against the wiles of the devil" (Ephesians 6: 11). The next verse says that "we do not wrestle against flesh and blood but against principalities, powers and rulers of darkness in this present age." Effective medical education is important to God's kingdom here on earth. The devil has been trying for many years to disrupt it. Those principalities, powers, and rulers of darkness will block us in any way they can.

When I first came to Purdue, I attended one of our departmental faculty meetings. We were a small group of seven people then. One of the other faculty members belittled me in front of all the others. Here I was, new to the department, trying to fit in, not yet understanding all the personal relationships in the group, and to be rejected and put down was extremely embarrassing. I had a great deal of difficulty with forgiveness for years. It was a huge problem for me especially since I was not attending church and had no deep spirituality. I remember complaining to God about the lack of inner peace. This was one of the factors that drove me back to church and into the charismatic movement. As the problem persisted, I tried to combat it with fasting and prayer. For about five years, I fasted one whole day a week, pleading with God for help with the situation. It gave me great relief, and eventually, this faculty member left Purdue, and I was grateful. I'm ashamed to say that I was less effective than I should have been in my work because of unforgivingness. This man returns to Purdue periodically, and now, our relationship is a cordial one.

My office is in the pharmacy building, and our medical classrooms are in the subbasement of the School of Veterinary Medicine on the Purdue University campus. So I show up at the vet school only for my lectures and am not around enough to get the feel of the entire spiritual atmosphere. However, my impression is the esprit de corps is good, and the dean is doing a fine job. The students are comfortable and work hard, and everyone seems happy. This is not a trivial thing since so many organizations are beset with problems. Yet our purposes there are of the highest importance in God's kingdom and a prime target for "evil principalities and powers."

I also teach a few labs to pharmacy students and, as I mentioned, am adviser to the Christian Pharmacy Student Association. We have some ten to twenty students out of about five hundred in our College of Pharmacy who attend our meetings. I'm grateful for each one. They are bright, strong young people who want to be the best pharmacists they can be. About 75 percent of young people stop going to church when they go to college. All our students go to church. We meet once a week to study the interface between pharmacy and Christianity. Our purpose is threefold, to bring each other closer to Christ, to develop close professional relationships in the group, and to learn how to deal with patients in a Christian manner.

There is so much sadness and so many health problems in our society today, a pharmacist with a positive Christian spirit can do much good. The pharmacist needs to be a kindly, parental figure and encouraging to all. This attitude is a corollary to a deep, convicted belief in the completeness of God's love and power and cannot be a superficial nicety. So a deep spirituality is needed by a pharmacist to provide the proper support for the patient. Thus, our Purdue Pharmacy Christian Student Association is important.

Seems to me there are two contrasting approaches to conducting a prayer group for Christian pharmacy students. One is charismatic with an open, welcoming (everybody hugs everybody else) attitude and based on the belief that Jesus is the salvation for each one of us. The other is cordial but proper and rather stiff. To me the former is fun and heartwarming. The latter is what we have in most mainline Christian churches. It serves a purpose but mostly deals with facts and is often just a cognitive experience.

Students can join our group during their prepharmacy years, so they may be with us for as many as four years. Thus we have a "rapid" turnover. When new students join our group, it takes a while for them to understand the depth of commitment to pharmacy and to Christianity that we have. So in the fall of the year, we are a bit disorganized especially if we have a new president who doesn't really have a good understanding either. We are ecumenical and so have spiritualities ranging from Pentecostal to that of the mainline churches. In my opinion, it's critical for the group to hear good, heartwarming testimonies early in the fall so the new students can be "indoctrinated" quickly.

One year, our indoctrination was not very effective, and we were divided into two camps, one favoring the charismatic and the other a formal approach. Things were stiff and awkward from the start. Our whole year was a roller-coaster ride. We had several bland, insipid meetings. But then, we had some guest speakers who did an outstanding job. They saved the year for us.

We invited Dr. Turek back, and he gave a profound overview of the concepts of divine healing. He mentioned that some healings are sudden, and others are slow in developing. He himself slipped on the ice one winter and that injury developed into a chronic hip inflammation that persisted for about a year. He couldn't sleep on the injured side. Then he went to a prayer meeting, and someone prayed for healing of an injured hip. Dr. Turek had not even mentioned his problem, but the healing took place immediately and the pain from the injury has not returned. When it happens to you, it convinces you of the reality of divine healing.

Dr. Turek also mentioned a church in Baghdad, Iraq—St. George's. It is an Anglican Christian Church, but many Muslims attend this church, and many healings have occurred there. A rear admiral of the US Navy who had been stationed in Iraq visited John Turek's home and told about a Muslim man who went to St. George's to pray for the healing of his daughter who was seriously ill in the hospital. The pastor there, Canon Andrew White, is a powerful man of God, and he also prayed for this man's daughter. So after Canon White prayed for her, he told him to go to the hospital because his daughter was being healed. It took him about two hours to get to the hospital, and when he got there, he was told that his daughter had died about an hour ago. He was overwhelmed with sorrow and confusion since he was told that his daughter was being healed, and he wept bitterly. He stood by his daughter lying on the bed with the sheet covering her face and, with deep sobs, reached over and pulled down the sheet and embraced her. Then he heard her say, "Daddy, I'm hungry, would you please get me something to eat?" How great is our God, and how strong is the power of his hand?

Another speaker was invited to our group to enhance the quality of our usual meetings. Greg Hockerman is a PhD in pharmacology and works in the same department at Purdue that I do. He was returning from vacation in Switzerland about ten years ago when a drunk driver ran a red light as Greg was leaving O'Hare Airport in Chicago. His van was struck, and two of his three children in the backseat died in the resulting fire. Greg tried desperately to save them and sustained severe burns on his head and arms. Can you imagine the anguish? Both he and his wife were devastated. How could this happen since he was such a fine Christian man? After this, Greg said he lost all interest in science and was considering resigning his position at Purdue. However, by the grace of God, he was able to continue as a faculty member and has been amazingly successful. He shared how both he and his wife suffered deep emotional pain. Instead of separating them, the pain actually drew them closer together. Dr. Hockerman's testimony was a strong witness to the power of God to help people who go through deep emotional trauma and still continue to be productive. Since pharmacists often get involved in the deeply emotional experiences of their patients, this sharing came at a critical time for the benefit of our Christian Pharmacy Student Group.

We were also blessed in this class to have a student from Nigeria who was a Spirit-filled, tongue-speaking Charismatic. His name was Osarodion Nosakhara, "Nosa." He was a very gracious, strong young man who made deeply insightful, spiritual statements in our meetings and was respectful to everyone. He volunteered to give five presentations to our group dealing with the interaction between pharmacy and our Christian faith. One of his presentations was entitled "Peaceoprolol," a hypothetical drug designed to bring peace in this troubled world of ours. It was a parody on the beta-blocking drug, propranolol. The presentation to our group was well-done and showed good insight into the relationship between pharmacy and Christianity. Nosa published this presentation in *Christianity and Pharmacy*, the official journal of Christian Pharmacists Fellowship International.

Nosa, along with Drs. Hockerman and Turek, was our salvation that year. Because of his participation in our group, Nosa received the Outstanding Member of a Purdue University Student Organization Award. He was selected from over one hundred students, and we deeply appreciated his contribution to PPCSA.

Why the roller coaster? People in our Christian Pharmacy Student Group come from different denominational backgrounds and have different degrees of spirituality. We would naturally differ in approaches to examine the relationships between pharmacy and Christianity. Nosa had a strong, Pentecostal approach. Others would prefer something more bland and not so Charismatic. It seems to me though that since pharmacy deals with serious health matters, we need something strong to combat the deception and the tricks of the devil. This is serious business; we can't be wishy-washy. Doubt was a great problem in Nazareth at the time of Christ. It is an equally great problem in modern times. Spiritual warfare is real and requires strong, committed people to handle it.

Unfortunately, the formal approach won out, and our meetings lost their charismatic quality. However, a new faculty member who is a committed Christian and has had extensive clinical pharmacy experience and a law degree as well joined our group. Missy Blue has done a fine job for us, and the group is thriving under her leadership. God knows what he is doing, so our group is still doing well and, hopefully, will continue to be a positive influence on pharmacy at Purdue and in the state of Indiana.

I'm indebted to the fine young students who have who have provided outstanding leadership for us. Jean Ann Custis Neese was president of our group for two years and was the one who had us officially recognized by Purdue University as a student organization. Erica (Uitto) Wheeler also did a fine job for us for three years and now practices pharmacy in the Minneapolis area. Creighton Kaiser was the son of a well-respected pharmacist. He greatly admired his father, and he himself was deeply committed to pharmacy, a straight-A student. He also was a committed Christian and shared that when he was on the high school football team, one of his teammates reprimanded him for taking the Lord's name in vain. It was a deep spiritual experience for him, and he mended his ways. So he was an ideal leader for us with good people skills and with a great love for pharmacy and deeply spiritual as well. We had quality meetings, and everything went smoothly when he was president for three years. Although women may have special spiritual insight, men have also made strong contributions to our group over the eighteen years of our existence.

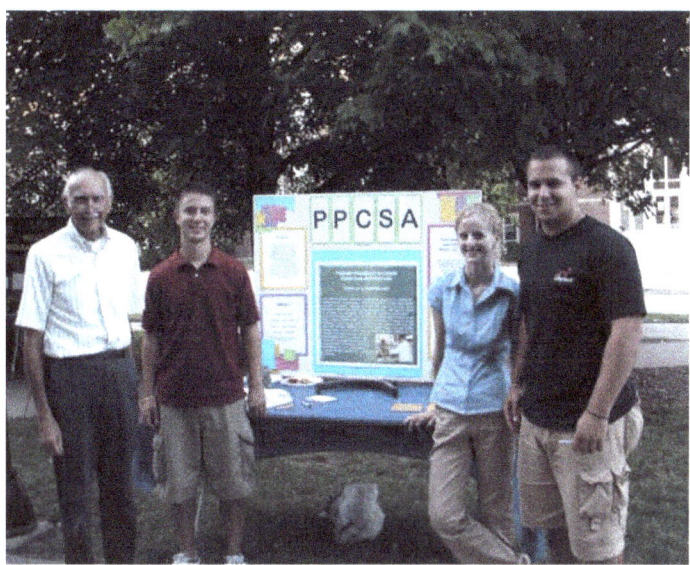

This is our Purdue Pharmacy Christian Student Association display at our "Pharmacy First Nighter" August 28, 2007 on the Mall in front of the Pharmacy College. From right to left are Creighton Kaiser, Jessica (Larva) Tribolletti and Cory Smith. All 3 served as President of our organization, Creighton for 3 years, Jessica for 1 and Cory for 2. All 3 did very well for us and we appreciated their competent help very much.

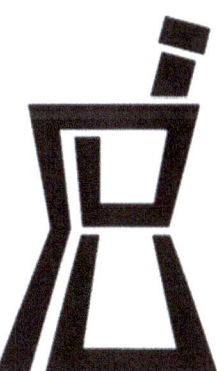

This is the College of Pharmacy official logo. We see a mortar and pestle. The mortar is shaped by the letters P and U standing for Purdue University. Our Christian Pharmacy Student Association modified the logo by including a cross in the mortar.

CHAPTER 7

Holy Spirit Power

He said to them, "Did you receive the Holy Spirit when you believed?"
And they said, "No, we have not even heard of the Holy Spirit."
—Acts 19:2

Paul was speaking in Acts to disciples in Ephesus. They were good Christians, but they had not so much as heard of the Holy Spirit. Today, all Christians have heard of the Holy Spirit, but many don't understand what that means. There are some churches where you're not welcome if you are Spirit-filled. They don't want you in their church. Some Christians don't know how essential it is to have the wisdom, strength, courage, and peace provided by the Holy Spirit. I've heard a middle-aged man ask whether we need to have a deep experience with the Holy Spirit to be a good Christian. Some people don't understand how important the Spirit is and what a dramatic change is needed for a person to allow themselves to be dominated by the Holy Spirit.

I believe the Holy Spirit was instrumental in the establishment of the United States of America. For George Washington and his band of ragged soldiers to defeat the most powerful army in the world was a miracle.

Washington was a godly man. He prayed for an hour every morning and also every night. He encouraged his men at Valley Forge to be righteous men like himself and to keep in mind the godly purpose of what they were doing. General Washington insisted on high moral standards and was able to maintain a good spirit among his troops even in the cold winter of Valley Forge.

Peaceful demonstrations and passive resistance, as used in India and South Africa, are powerful ways to obtain people's rights but were unknown in George Washington's time. General Washington had the responsibility to forcibly resist the tyranny of King George of England, and he did so in a humane manner. The battle of Trenton, New Jersey, was a major event in the Revolutionary War, involving about three thousand men, yet the number of lives lost was minimal. This was a tribute to the American leadership and reflects guidance by the Holy Spirit.

Washington led his soldiers in an attack on British German mercenaries at Christmastime in Trenton. On Christmas night, he and his men crossed the Delaware River to surprise the German garrison there on the morning of December 26, 1777. It was raining and started to sleet, which turned to snow. Large flat barges carried the horses and cannon, but the troops were transported in boats. Miraculously, no one was lost in the crossing, which involved about 1,500 men. The British warned the German colonel Ralls of an impending attack, but the colonel thought that a brief skirmish earlier with some local insurgents was the end of it. Washington was upset about the small battle, thinking that it would forewarn the Germans, but it didn't. Colonel Ralls didn't even send out patrols that night because of the bad weather. Thus, the Germans were not well prepared for the attack, and Washington had a good plan to prevent escape of any of the Hessians. All toll the Germans lost only twenty-two men, including colonel Ralls, but about one thousand were captured. So Washington won a great victory for the Colonial army. It was a turning point for the conflict.

Washington was filled with fervor for the righteous cause of the war. The future and the religious freedom of the colonies were at stake. The dreams of the Patriots were being threatened. Were they going to have a democracy with liberty and justice for all, or were they going to have the tyranny so common in other countries?

As a godly man, Washington was a great leader for the soldiers in his army and also was outstanding as first president of the United States. People wanted to make him king, but he refused! He said that this country was to be special and that religious freedom was to be given priority. He wasn't thinking of himself, and I believe the Holy Spirit guided him.

We have a precious religious heritage here in the United States. We have freedom here, and we know that freedom is not free. Many men had to die so that we can enjoy the privileges of democracy in this country. The signers of the Declaration of Independence knew that by signing they would die if the British won. Yet they risked their lives anyway. One of the signers was rejected by his neighbors who were loyal to the British, and he soon passed away. Many Holy Spirit—led people have sacrificed their ambitions and even their own lives so that we can have a free country. I've lived in England and Switzerland and have visited China, Mexico, Canada, France, Germany, Israel, Taiwan, Holland, and the Philippines, but nowhere have I experienced the freedom we have in the USA. Please forgive my bias for my homeland and understand that each of the countries that I visited has special advantages and something good to offer its citizens.

I remember a Purdue student in our Christian Pharmacy Group ask, "What does the Holy Spirit have to do with my personal testimony?" I was so surprised I didn't know what to say. It took my breath away. How could a member of our group ask such a question? It broke my heart. But it is not uncommon for members of Christian churches to fail to understand the workings of the Holy Spirit.

Once I shared my own baptism in the Holy Spirit with a pastor and another Christian man in a counseling session. The baptism was a deep, meaningful experience to me, something precious to my soul. I thought it was appropriate since we were talking about relationships. The pastor asked why I wanted to share my story with them. I answered that I wanted to tell them where I was coming from to illustrate the power of the Holy Spirit. It seemed to me that even the pastor did not really understand the absolute importance of the Holy Spirit. The other man also appeared bewildered by the story of my baptism at the age of forty-two years. I was accused of being a fanatic and waving my pocket Bible around, saying, "There is only one way to salvation." I don't remember saying that, but it is true that there is only one way, and the Holy Spirit is an important part of it.

Billy Graham claims he didn't have a deep sudden experience with the Holy Spirit, but in one of his books, he tells a story of himself as a young man. He had a girlfriend he was very fond of, and how he cried when she told him he was not spiritual enough and she didn't want to see him anymore. It seems to me that this was his baptism in the Holy Spirit. God had to allow for Billy's heart to be broken so that the good

Lord himself could enter into the deep recesses there and occupy the throne of Billy's life. We are so stubborn; we insist on being in charge and running things our own way.

Once I tried to share my charismatic approach to Christianity with a friend at church. He was an unusual fellow but seemed to be open to my comments at first. I suggested he read the Gospel of Mark, the shortest of all Gospels. A fast-moving, exciting story. It took him a year to do it. I knew then he really didn't take me seriously. People used to a certain way don't want to change. Resistance to the Holy Spirit can be strong.

For an organization, large or small, to be effective for God, the Holy Spirit has to be allowed to work. Those who have executive control must realize this and allow him to direct the group in the right way. The four organizations I have been most closely associated with are all very important godly groups of people with serious divine purposes. May I comment briefly on the involvement of the Holy Spirit in each of these organizations? The health of people involved correlates with the quality of the organization, so these comments are pertinent to the purpose of this book (i.e., to correlate spirituality and health).

Nearly sixty years ago, I came to Purdue to get a graduate degree in pharmacology. Glen Jenkins was dean, and he had built up a fine research institution. He was a positive thinker and proud of the people he had trained for pharmaceutical research. There was a good spirit here. When I returned to Purdue in 1969, there was still a good spirit here and a healthy research atmosphere. My boss, Dr. Tom Miya, actually encouraged me to go to church. He was a godly man and a good pharmacologist. However, the political atmosphere was not favorable, and he began to have gastrointestinal problems and left Purdue to assume the deanship of the Pharmacy School at North Carolina. Dr. Roger Maickel took Dr. Miya's place. Dr. Maickel was well trained in Dr. Bernard Brodie's lab at NIH and was an outstanding leader for us in pharmacology at Purdue. But again because of politics, he had to step down and died a few years later. He was a fine Catholic man, and it broke my heart. George Yim became chairman and did a good job but had no good spiritual base and lasted only a few years. He retired, and the department disintegrated and was taken over by medicinal chemistry.

Actually, this change was a blessing. Twenty years later, ours is the strongest research department on the Purdue campus. Under the leadership of Rick Borch, MD, PhD, we have expanded to twenty-five faculty members. The old Department of Pharmacology had only seven members, and we struggled getting grant money. The chemists had an advantage over us. They could offer the enticement of making a new drug for curing a disease while pharmacology was generally concerned with side effects and mechanisms of existing drugs. Dr. Gary Isom (principal investigator) and I (coinvestigator) had continual NIH grant support for twenty-five years, working on toxic mechanisms of cyanide. This chemical has caused more acute human deaths than any other chemical has. It is still important since death by smoke inhalation often involves cyanide generated by heating plastic. Even so, chemists generally have the advantage, and we have had faculty from our department make clinically useful drugs for AIDS and for parkinsonism. I didn't want our pharmacology department combined with medicinal chemistry, but I can see how God guided Dean Charles Rutledge and Dr. Rick Borch (chairman of the combined departments) to develop something truly outstanding for our college of pharmacy.

Dr. Maickel brought with him a young faculty member from pharmacology at Indiana University Medical School at Bloomington. Joe Zabic had his office next to mine, and we became good friends. He too was Catholic but was not deeply spiritual and passed away with a heart attack at the age of fifty-one. He and I used to go to the church together. I still miss him although he died twenty years ago. I tried to encourage him to read the Bible more, but he wasn't interested. I'm thinking he'd still be here if he had joined our fellowship.

Purdue is a secular university, but fortunately, our dean, Craig Svensson, is a godly man, and our Pharmacy College is among the most outstanding in the USA. I believe there is a correlation between our dean's godly orientation and the quality of our college.

Our Lafayette Center for Medical Education is about forty years old, and we have had some outstanding students go through our program. We are building a new facility, but now, we are located in a subbasement of Purdue School of Veterinary Medicine. We have a fine program, and our students do well on the board exams, but it takes a great effort both on the part of the faculty as well as the students. Even so, there is some stress involved. In the winter, we're all jammed together in a small room, and colds are common, and seasonal affective disorder causes some absenteeism, but our attendance overall is excellent. Where there is a godly atmosphere with kindness and respect, good health prevails.

When the Holy Spirit dominates a group of people, it is a heartwarming, exciting thing. Everyone feels welcome, and there is joy, and all present have a good time. That magic spiritual ingredient brings people together and allows Christian love to flow freely. Our Sunday school program at Blessed Sacrament is a good one, and people are congenial and respectful to one another. Some of the teachers exude love, and it's a joy to observe this in their classes. What a feeling of health it brings. The Holy Spirit allows for an openness but also calls for order in the classroom. Then classes can flow easily, and everyone benefits from a joyful, well-ordered lesson.

I once went to a retirement party for a man who had worked for various Catholic elementary schools all his life. I first met him when he gave a speech about thirty-five years earlier. He had gone to the seminary for a while but dropped out. He made up a slide show of his career and showed it at the retirement party. He coached softball, soccer, football, and track teams and said how he enhanced the spirituality of his students. I have no doubt that he made an effort in the right direction and did much good in his career. I had the feeling though that he could have done much more if he had allowed the Holy Spirit to fully direct his efforts. Only when we have a deep experience with the Holy Spirit and allow him to guide our lives are we able to make a strong contribution to building the church here on earth. I know I've fallen short in my own efforts to serve him, and it was only after I had been baptized in the Holy Spirit that I was able to forget myself and to do at least some things worthwhile for the kingdom.

Many of us are like St. John the Apostle, who, with his brother James, was one of the sons of thunder, very aggressive and outgoing without much understanding or compassion. When he was young, he was the one who asked Christ if he should call down fire and brimstone on the Samaritans when they refused hospitality to Jesus and his apostles. Later in life, St. John learned the great value of love balanced with compassion and understanding. This is especially evident in the third chapter of his first epistle. My hope is that we all learn to incorporate the Holy Spirit into our life's work as St. John did and to minimize the influence of our own egos.

CHAPTER 8

Importance of Humility

Be kind to one another because most of us are fighting a hard battle.
—Ian Maclaren

People are generally respectful to those who have special abilities and authority over them—the clergy, physicians, pharmacists, dentists, nurses, teachers, elected officials, etc. They know that these powerful figures can be of great benefit to them. These people have an understanding and training to help others in their need. These authority figures should also respect the people they serve. They should even step off their pedestals and show that they love those they serve and take responsibility for them.

In his book on mirth, Father James Martin, SJ, mentions Pope John XXIII as an exemplar of humility ("Between Heaven and Mirth" Harper/Collins Publishers 2011, New York, NY). A little boy asked the pope's advice. He couldn't decide whether to be a policeman or the pope. Pope John replied, "Dear Bruno, if you want my advice, be a policeman for that cannot be improvised." Then he added that anybody can be pope; look at me. It's no wonder he was such a beloved, cherished leader. He could bend down to meet that little boy and encourage him on the way he should go.

In his book *Spirituality in Patient Care* (Templeton Press, 2007, W. Conshohocken, PA), Harold Koenig, MD, mentions how important it is for a doctor to relate to his patient. He says if the doctor's patient is a little girl, and she asks him to evaluate the health of her teddy bear, he needs to take out his stethoscope and perform an examination. He has to make the most of the opportunity to meet the needs of his patient.

There is a delicate balance between respect and overfamiliarity. To be a godly person and effective for God's purposes, we each need the help of the Holy Spirit. Those who have any authority should use it to express their love and care for others. All authority does come from God (Romans 13:1), and he can use it to build his kingdom here on earth.

"Pomposity is a danger when you are perceived to have power over people," says Father Jim Martin, SJ. How heartwarming it is when people in authority can bring themselves down to the level of others and truly help them as a fellow human being. After all, we're on this life journey together. We need each other. Doctors and pharmacists need their patients as much as the patients need them.

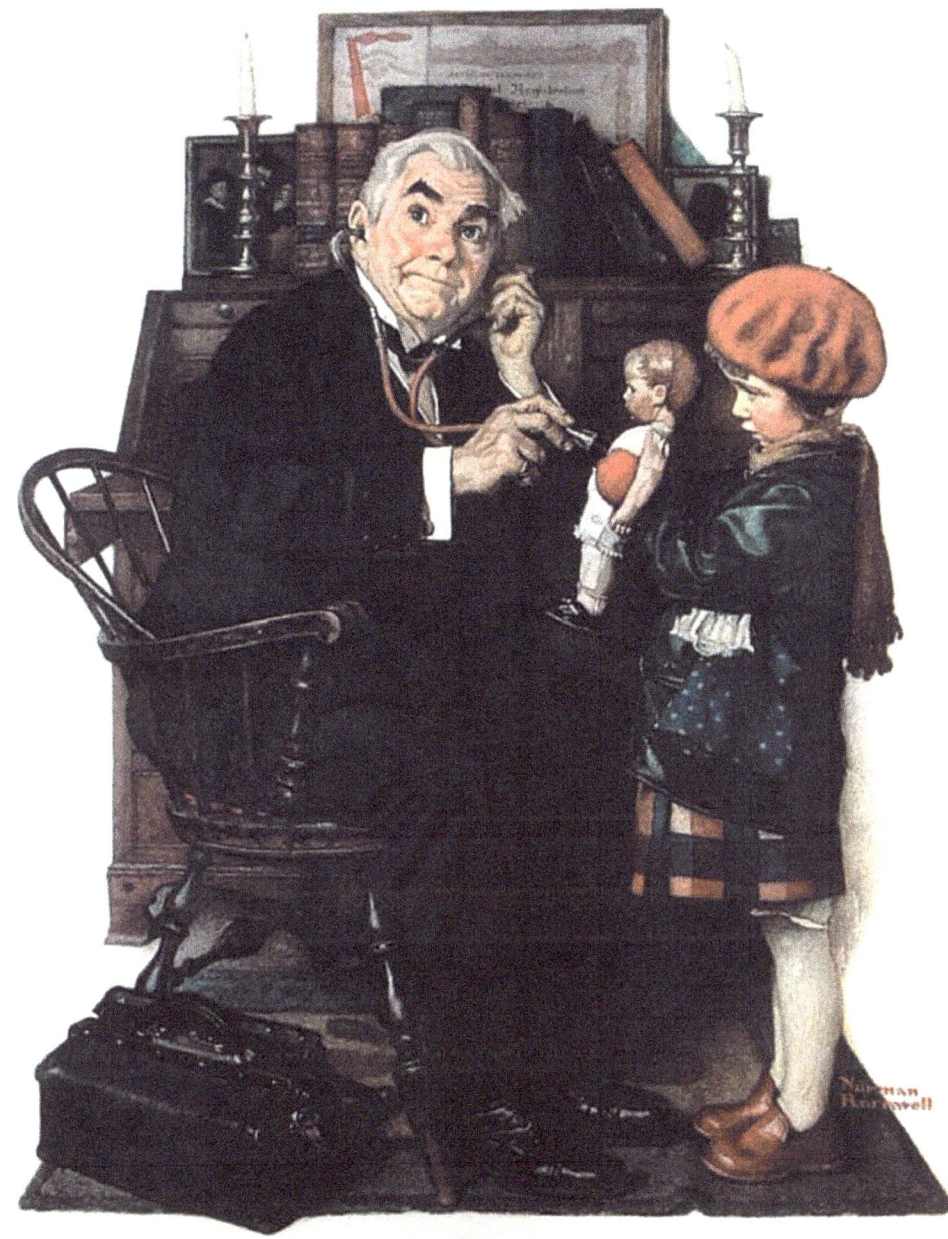

"The Doctor and the Doll" by Norman Rockwell was on the cover of "The Saturday Evening Post" in 1929. He beat Harold Koenig by almost a hundred years. A heartwarming picture showing good social sensitivity on the part of the physician.

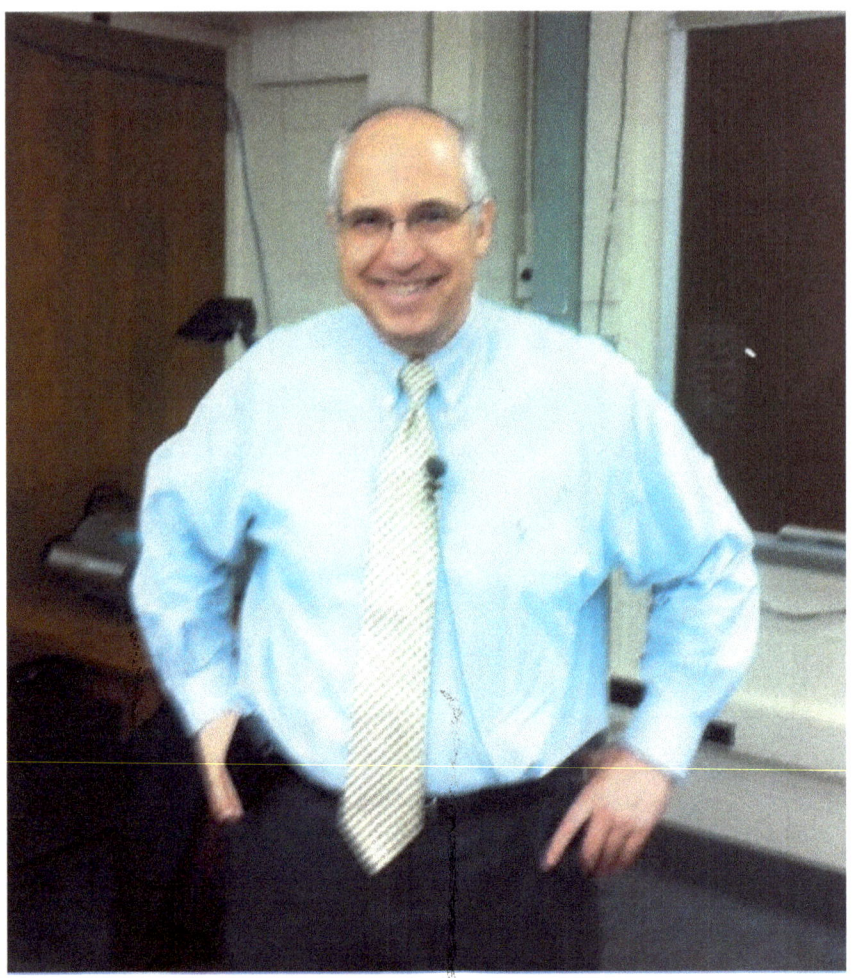

Each fall we have a Faculty Retreat prior to the beginning of the semester. A few years ago Dr Adi Haramati from the Department of Physiology at Georgetown University School of Medicine shared his philosophy in teaching medical students. He explained how he tried to encourage and guide these young students and to foster curiosity in them. He even had a session in which he taught us all to relax. The lights were turned down and he had us sit comfortably in our chairs while he had us repeat over and over "My arms are relaxed and warm; My legs are relaxed and warm; My abdomen is relaxed; My head is refreshed and cool". To learn effectively, the students need to have a relaxed attitude and develop that equanimity characteristic of good physicians.

CHAPTER 9

Outstanding Health Personnel

Prayer and good humor are two of the strongest alternative medicines.
—Joe Hurt, MD, PhD

Shannon Oates is a fine physician and also a really good teacher at our Lafayette Center for Medical Education. Her daughters were in my Sunday school class. Dr. Oates sat in on my class one Sunday in which we were to discuss divine healing. I was a little apprehensive because I didn't know her attitude toward this whole concept. So I asked her before class if she believed in divine healing. She said, "It happens all the time." Also, she said, "It makes me look good when God heals the patient." This lady is an outstanding physician and very successful and appreciates the importance of a godly, faith-filled attitude in the healing process. No wonder she is such a helpful, popular clinician and an asset to her community.

Bernie Seigel, MD, is a surgeon at Yale New Haven Hospital. He deals with many cancer patients and has noticed the importance of a positive, hopeful attitude on the part of the patient in the outcome of medical problems. Even with the most dire prognosis, some patients survive. Dr.

Siegel found that the ones who do survive are those with a good outlook on life and a strong desire to live. He mentions in his book (*Love, Medicine and Miracles*, Harper, New York, 1986) one cancer patient to whom he was explaining the importance of the will to live. The patient's wife was present also. The wife said, "Oh, Dr. Siegel, my husband wants to live." The patient then commented that he really did not want to live. He said he remembers his father who was a fine, intelligent man. The son loved and admired his father and looked up to him. Then his father got Alzheimer's disease and couldn't even remember his own name. The patient said, "My cancer is serious and that's fine with me. I don't want to be like my father. I'll just go now and avoid all the problems." It's difficult to bring about a healing in a patient with a negative attitude like this man had.

Dr. Siegel also mentions a patient with a split personality. As in the movie *Three Faces of Eve*, people can switch between different personalities rapidly. The woman, Eve, was a poor, self-effacing farmwife normally but could change in an instant to an outgoing swinger. Anyway, Dr. Siegel noted that a man had type 2 diabetes with one of his personalities, but with another of his personalities, there was no diabetes. Amazing how the same physical being could have an illness with one of his personalities but not with the other.

Sir William Osler (1849-1919) was one of the greatest physicians of his day and made many contributions to the practice of medicine. His father was an Anglican missionary to Canada, and Dr. Osler was the youngest of nine children. He too wanted to be a minister early on but decided instead to go into medicine. He graduated from the University of Toronto and became a faculty member at Johns Hopkins. He, along with some other professors there, developed that medical school into one of the finest in the world. Dr. Osler became world famous by writing a popular textbook of medicine. These men were expert clinicians also. In those days, if you were very ill and wanted to be healed, you went to Johns Hopkins. The quality of treatment there is still outstanding today. Dr. Osler realized in those days (early 1900s) that drugs did not change the prognosis of diseases. They were only palliative, relieving symptoms, so drugs were used sparingly by Dr. Osler. Great emphasis was placed on high-quality nursing care. Dr. Osler practiced medicine according to the high standards of the Hippocratic oath. He had such good rapport with the patients that they felt better when he walked into the room. He believed that a calm even spirit was the greatest asset of a physician. How fortunate were Dr. Osler's students to be exposed not only to his wisdom but also to his positive, hopeful attitude toward his patients.

Dr. William Osler left Johns Hopkins to become chairman of the Department of Medicine at Oxford University in England. He had married the granddaughter of Paul Revere, and they had one son. So they moved to England. His contributions there were recognized by the British government, and he was knighted by the king of England. His son was a pilot in World War I and was killed action. It broke Sir William Osler's heart, and he died soon after.

A contemporary of Dr. Osler was Sigmund Freud (1856-1939), an Austrian neurologist trained at the University of Vienna who also studied in Paris. He is credited with establishing psychoanalysis as a medical specialty. Prior to that time, mental illness was thought to be an organic disease. Dr. Freud showed that some mental problems can be caused by unhealthy thoughts and can be treated by counseling. This was a tremendous breakthrough in our approach to the problems of mental illness. It's obvious to us now but was revolutionary in the days of Dr. Freud. Thank God for the scientific insight of this man.

Of all physicians, Dr. Albert Schweitzer, MD (1875-1965), certainly knew the value of high ethical standards. He was an ordained Lutheran minister and a PhD in philosophy prior to entering medical school at the University of Strasbourg. He thoroughly understood the importance of the Hippocratic oath, and I believe it contributed to his outstanding success. He gave up a lucrative medical practice in Paris, France, to become a missionary in Lamborene, French Equatorial Africa, on the Agobe River.

It was a very difficult experience for Dr. Schweitzer. The heat and humidity in Equatorial Africa (now Gabon) are intense. However, Dr. Schweitzer was noted for his pleasant disposition. The staff at the clinic ate meals together, and the mealtime was a great joy to nurses and physicians alike. Dr. Schweitzer was a godly man, and his kindness was a positive factor for the patients as well as the medical staff there in Africa.

Dr. Schweitzer spoke strongly against prejudice of any kind and wrote a book, *Reverence for Life*. He used much of his own wealth to expand his mission in Lamborene to seventy buildings equivalent to a five-hundred-bed hospital. He lived by principles given in the oath of Hippocrates. He received the Nobel Peace Prize in 1952.

Although pharmacists generally don't become as famous as physicians, they are nevertheless very important in the care of sick people. Gallup polls done through the years reveal that the pharmacist is the most respected of all professionals. Pharmacists are readily available to patients and are knowledgeable and helpful in answering health and drug-related questions. In preparing my lectures, I frequently call pharmacists at the local hospitals and drugstores, I deeply appreciate their help. They know which drugs are most popular and most useful. A deep spirituality greatly enhances the helpfulness and effectiveness of pharmacists as well as doctors.

Walter Cronkite, the anchor on *CBS Evening News* for many years, tells of his grandfather who was a pharmacist and owned a drugstore in Leavenworth, Kansas (*Catholic Digest*, September 2006). As a boy, Walter worked for his grandfather and greatly respected him. When he was older and a little hard of hearing, Mr. Fritsche got a job helping out in a chain pharmacy. When Walter returned from covering the postwar Nuremburg Trials, the manager of the chain store asked to talk to him. He explained that he wanted to fire his grandfather after he was there a week. Whenever the phone would ring, Mr. Fritsche would shush the whole store so he could hear. The manager thought it would drive away business, but the opposite happened. People began to eavesdrop on Mr. Fritsche's calls. "He'd get calls demanding all kinds of advice, and the whole store would listen quietly to the answers. When he'd hang up, everybody would be smiling at everybody else. They were amused at the old fellow, of course, but they were raking in some of his advice too, and they sort of relaxed." The manager said he never got a chance to say these things to Mr. Fritsche before he died, so he wanted to tell Mr. Cronkite and express his thankfulness for his grandfather's help. Because there is usually no charge for patient counseling and pharmacists are readily available, they provide much needed advice for patients in health matters. A positive, faith-filled attitude is a great asset to the professional practice of pharmacy.

Edward Fredrichs, MD, was a student at Northwestern University Medical School at the time I was studying there for the PhD in pharmacology.

Dr. Fredrichs trained in internal medicine in Minneapolis but switched to psychosomatic practice when he recognized the importance of the brain-body connection and how the mind influences health and disease. Soldiers in battle become terribly frightened to the extent that they are paralyzed. They can't fire their weapons, nor can they run away. More common examples of psychosomatic actions are blushing, sweating, sighing, crying, and laughing. Diabetics have sudden changes in blood sugar and appetite due to psychophysiological effects, and arterial constriction, inflammation, or clotting may occur in other patients. Thoughts have a powerful effect on the health of the body.

Dr. Fredrichs recognized sleep as an important psychosomatic health factor. Two-thirds of his patients had sleep problems. Patients develop back problems when they don't sleep well for a period of several months. They live in a constant state of muscle tension. Surgery is sometimes required. Unfortunately, there are no good drugs for inducing a physiological sleep. Melatonin is a naturally occurring chemical produced by our pineal gland, which lies deep within the center of the brain. It produces a mild hypnotic effect but may cause some grouchiness and worsens autoimmune problems. Benzodiazepines like Ambien and especially barbiturates interfere with rapid eye movement (REM) sleep and, therefore, do not allow for a deep, restful experience. Some amnesia also occurs with Ambien, so Dr. Fredrichs uses low doses of benzodiazepines to obtain as good a quality of sleep as possible.

In the late '70s and early '80s, abuse of cocaine became popular, and Dr. Fredrichs found these addicts had terrible sleep problems. Abuse of other drug substances like alcohol, tobacco, and heroin similarly cause poor sleep. Furthermore, cocaine patients are secretive, don't feel good about themselves, and are poor communicators. It's difficult to interact with them. Dr. Fredrichs teaches his students to be persistent and maintain communication so they can be of some help to their addicted patients.

According to Dr. Fredrichs, a common cause of poor health is bad psychosocial interactions. Who would guess that these everyday human interactions are a factor in your own personal health? Your lifespan may be shortened by unpleasant relationships with those around you. We need the help of physicians and pharmacists as well as the help of the Holy Spirit not only to heal our physical ailments but also to help us forgive and love those around us.

Once a week, I memorize ten verses from the Psalms. In my fifth time through the 150 psalms, I'm now on number 119, the longest chapter in the Bible. I've discovered that this chapter is directly pertinent to personal interactions. Maybe that's why it's the longest chapter of all because personal interactions so commonly cause problems. People do all kinds of things to upset us. Psalm 119 reminds us over and over that we must focus on God's commandments, statutes, and precepts and not on other people.

Psalm 119 is also a healing psalm. "Let your tender mercies come to me that I may live; for your law is my delight" (verse 77). What a joy to know that his tender mercies continually flow into us. Also verse 71, "It is good that I have been afflicted that I may learn your statutes." There's a purpose to all this suffering. Furthermore, there is also this verse, "Unless your law had been my delight, I would have perished in my affliction" (verse 92). Thus, delighting in his law is an antidote to our afflictions. And in verse 107, "I am afflicted very much; revive me O Lord, according to your word." Even when our afflictions are great, his Word can revive us. Praise the Lord!

Dr. Fredrichs was recognized as a distinguished alumnus of Northwestern Medical School and rightfully so. He discovered novel insights into medical problems and taught his students to persevere in seeking relationships and to be especially kind to patients who have addiction problems and desperately need help.

CHAPTER 10

Humor and Healing

It would be helpful for the physician to have a stock of good honest stories to make patients laugh.

—John Ardurne

In 1964, forty-nine-year-old Norman Cousins, editor of the *Saturday Review*, an important literary magazine, was asked to be chairman of a conference in Moscow involving distinguished literary people from all over the world. This was a time when the Cold War was at its peak, so the meeting had political as well as literary significance. In July, Cousins flew to Moscow and essentially lost a night's sleep in the process. To his dismay, his hotel in Moscow had construction going on next door, and heavy machinery worked through the night. Furthermore, it was a hot July in Moscow, and there was no air-conditioning in the hotel, so Cousins had to open the windows at night, which allowed exhaust from the heavy machinery to come into his room. This went on through the entire week of the meeting and added to the stress of the situation. The conference went well, however, and Cousins returned home but, in doing so, lost another night's sleep.

It's not surprising that when Cousins arrived in the USA, he became seriously ill. He was hospitalized with ankylosing spondylitis (inflammation of the spine, joints, and ligaments). He was in constant, severe pain and could not even move his thumb without extreme discomfort. He could not sleep and lay awake all night on several successive nights. They gave him high doses of aspirin, which alone could make a person sick. A neurologist came by and gave a poor prognosis, saying Cousins had one chance in five hundred to survive.

Red cells in an anticoagulated blood sample settle only a few millimeters, if at all, in an hour's time in normal people. However, in patients with cancer, infection, inflammation, etc., sedimentation rate increases to about 70/hr. due to abnormal large proteins, which bind to the red cells. Cousins's sedimentation rate was 88.

Knowing that the large doses of aspirin they were giving him were of no benefit, Cousins checked himself out of the hospital with the help of his personal physician and into a motel room. He hired people to help him and rented funny movies and TV programs (Abbott and Costello, Laurel and Hardy, *Candid Camera*, etc.) and found that he could sleep for about two hours after watching these funny films. His sedimentation rate went down five millimeters with the laughter associated with viewing these films followed by periods of restful sleep. The decrease in sedimentation rate was cumulative when the procedure was repeated over and over, and after eight days, Cousins was able to move his thumb without pain. The decrease in sedimentation rate was an objective measure of the healing effect of laughter and sleep on Cousins's ankylosing spondylitis. Continuing this process, Cousins slowly recovered and returned to work after a few months. After a few years, he was able to play golf again with no pain. Cousins said he had no doubt that he would recover despite the grim prognosis by the neurologist. This was important in his survival. He thought a positive, hopeful attitude was critical for his eventual recovery. This remarkable story of the healing effect of laughter on a serious physical problem is recorded in Cousins' book *Anatomy of an Illness* (Bantum Books Inc. New York, 1979).

Bernie Siegel, MD, the surgeon, also claims that humor has a positive effect on the healing process. He goes further to say that exercise and play have effects similar to laughter. People with stiff personalities who cannot let themselves laugh and play are the ones who are not healed. He also describes the hearty, healing type of laughter (excluding nervous social laughter, which is so common) as "internal jogging." As jogging is good for your health so is a good belly laugh.

When adults are sick, they become like little kids again, according to Leslie Gibson, BS, RN. They need to be treated as such. She claims humor is a powerful therapeutic tool. She is a graduate of Purdue University School of Nursing and has a successful practice in a hospice in the Florida Suncoast and specializes in stress management and humor development. Her clients include Case Western Hospital and the US Department of Defense. She tries to bring humor into the hospital-type situation to counteract the "poor-me syndrome" and advocates clown training for volunteers. One of her favorites is a talking box, which repeats over and over, "Help, let me out of here." One of her practical jokes was to glue a coffee cup to the top of her car. This also gave rise to many funny situations. Leslie Gibson says the shortest distance between two people is laughter and suggests that health professionals ask patients who their favorite comedian is. Often they will answer and share one of their favorite jokes as well.

Leslie Gibson has worked extensively with Patch Adams. If you've seen the movie, you know how Patch tried to bring humor into hospital situations and how effective it was. Mrs. Gibson also maintains that there is a place for the healing power of humor in modern medical practice especially in a hospital setting.

Patch Adams, MD, made famous by the movie, is a popular speaker and is known as the "clown prince of physicians." He says fun has strong, beneficial effects especially in arthritis and mental health problems. He claims that hospitals are places of seriousness and solemnity and that such an atmosphere does not promote healing.

Sir William Osler, arguably one of the most effective physicians to come out of this part of the world, appreciated the medical benefits of humor. He made the statement that laughter is the music of life. He also indicated that you can keep yourself young with laughter. Humor was also critical for Albert Schweitzer and his staff as well as his patients. In those days, in Equatorial Africa, there were only two automobiles within a twenty-five-mile radius around the clinic at Lamborene. Wouldn't you know those two autos collided as they drove along the jungle pathways? Dr. Schweitzer had to treat both drivers for minor injuries. I'm sure this event provided for much hilarity at the clinic along the Agobe River. Even Dr. Sigmund Freud, as stern as he appears in his photographs, believed that humor is effective therapy although he probably did not realize that both psychological and physical problems respond to laughter.

Jack Hinson served as pastor of a Baptist church for several years and then was asked to be chaplain in C. J. Harris Regional Hospital in North

Carolina. After serving as chaplain for eighteen months, he became depressed with all the unhappiness and seriousness of medical and psychological problems endemic to the hospital scene. He saw a need for a joyful spirit, and he made an effort to bring some humor into that environment. After fourteen years' experience as chaplain, he wrote a book entitled *Laughter Was God's Idea* (Catch the Spirit of Appalachia, Western North Carolina, 2009). Chaplain Hinson believes God does have a sense of humor. Remember the story of Abraham and Sarah. Chaplain Jack tells of how they laughed when God informed them they were going to have a son. It was really funny. Abraham was one hundred and Sarah was ninety when Isaac was born. You usually don't see any bassinets in nursing homes. What a joke it was! Yet Abraham did indeed become the father of many nations. Nothing is impossible with God.

One story the chaplain told is of a patient who was informed she had cancer and had only six months to live. The chaplain told her to move to Cleveland. She asked if that would make her live longer. He said no, but it will seem longer. They both had a good laugh. Jack Hinson visited another eighty-two-year-old patient dying of cancer and asked how things were going. She said she was just muddling along. Jack mentioned he had just read Isaiah 40:31 and said if Isaiah were here, he would include her in his message. "They that wait upon the Lord will renew their strength, mount up with wings as eagles, run and not be weary, walk and not faint, and if they are sick, they shall keep muddling along." The lady laughed out loud and said she was glad she might be included in the Bible. Maybe Chaplain Hinson is right; maybe God did create laughter for a holy purpose. Only human beings have the gift of laughter. So far, as we know, animals do not have the capacity to appreciate humor as human beings do.

If humor is such a good, healthy thing, why don't we see more of it in churches? Father James Martin, SJ, in his book *Between Heaven and Mirth*, has a whole chapter on "Why so gloomy?" Why are Christians usually so serious? Father Martin quotes Barbara Ehrenreich, saying, that there is, in part, a historical explanation. In early European society, high-spirited gatherings (parties) were suppressed by authorities since they often involved "poking fun at civic and church leaders, thus posing a threat to social order." What a shame that we have inherited this attitude. Father Martin admits however, that many saints had a keen sense of humor.

Thank God, also, that many pastors are happy, humorous people. We had a Franciscan priest, Father Sylvester Hepner, who would have the people rolling in the aisles with laughter on Sunday mornings. He told one about the three ministers who were discussing how they divided up the Sunday collection. The first said that his way was easy; he just draws a line on the ground and takes the collection and throws it up. Whatever falls on one side of the line is for God's work; whatever falls on the other side was for his own personal use. The second said that he did something similar and draws a circle. He throws the Sunday collection up, and whatever falls within the circle is for God's work and the rest is for his own use. The last minister said he did something different, that he just throws the collection up, and whatever God catches he can have. Everyone felt better after listening to Father Sylvester's sermons. The church was always packed. What a blessing he was. But overall, humor is probably not the main reason why churchgoers live longer than other people, but it helps.

Harvy Cox mentions in a 1984 article in the *Boston Globe* that Dante, in his *Divine Comedy* reports he heard laughter as he approached the celestial sphere of heaven. Apparently, God laughs because he "knows how it all turns out in the end." Cox suggests that "there is something genuinely comic about Easter. Could it be that laughter is God's answer to those who derided God's Son and who continue to hound God's followers today?" Holy laughter may be a gift and a defense against despair for "God's gentle people" (*The Joyful Christ: The Healing Power of Humor* by Cal Samra, Harper, San Francisco, 1986).

Dr. William Kirk Kilpatrick on the faculty at Boston College, in his book (*Psychological Seduction: The Failure of Modern Psychology*, Roger A. McCaffery Publishers, Ridgefield, CT, 1983) says that psychology has become too serious. Any remarks made are often overanalyzed. The psychologist tries to separate individuals and keep them apart from others and this precludes laughter. These people rarely laugh since laughing requires self-abandonment. Good humor is founded on an ability to reach out and understand other people. Sometimes laughter is useful and can destroy evil without malice. Christ's laughter comes from one who has been betrayed by friends and felt the touch of the torturer.

In her book, Rhonda Beaman suggests that the part of humor that has healing properties is mirth (*You're Only Young Twice*, Vanderwyk and Burnham, 2006). The other two parts of humor, the wit and the laughter, probably, are not as effective. Wit may be sarcastic, and laughter can occur when nothing is really funny. The nervous social laughter which is so common is usually not associated with a feeling of mirth. That deep down, good feeling of mirth and joy is the healing factor according to Dr. Beaman. She mentions that people with heart disease are 40 percent less likely to laugh when something funny happens and suggests we all need to maintain the playfulness and joy we had as children.

CHAPTER 11

Importance of Fellowship and Teamwork

Flaming enthusiasm, backed by common horse sense and persistence, is the quality which most frequently makes for success.

—Dale Carnegie

We mentioned the need for doctors to stop being cowboys and to become pit crew people. This is not an easy task. Human relationships are so complex, and we all have natural affinities. There are certain people we are naturally attracted to. However, in my opinion, there is just one really attractive feature in each one of us. We are each attractive according to the degree we are Christlike. Yes, there are physical features, common interests, shared likes and dislikes, similar attitudes, etc., which are important in relationships, but it's that genuine, Christlike goodness that radiates from a person that really makes them attractive. You can tell when a person has that true joy deep in their hearts. Those really good people are all the same. You enjoy just being around them. They reach out to others, they encourage others, they are compassionate, they are generous, and they are the salt of the earth. Fellowship and teamwork are of critical importance in the medical profession. We, in the medical area, need to have that deep, genuine, loving, godly attitude toward other people.

No matter what profession we're in, we need to deal with people, and having good fellowship benefits us all. Jonathan and David in the Old Testament were good friends despite their contrasting backgrounds. David was a shepherd boy, and Jonathan was a king's son, yet their relationship was a godly thing and a blessing to the community as they looked out for one another and tried to be helpful. There is a great need today for strong, godly relationships between people to strengthen our society; genuine, pure, deeply spiritual friendships which would benefit our communities. Too many people think only of themselves and ignore others. The word *idiot* is derived from the Greek word *idiotes*, which means "someone who thinks only of himself."

A few years ago, a speaker addressed our medical faculty and told of a group of medical students who agreed to work together in studying for the Medical National Board Exams Step 1. They were not the best students in the class, but they had good relationships, and they each worked hard and helped and encouraged one another. They would share the work, and each would examine different topics and share with one another what they learned. The results were amazing. This group of ordinary students achieved some of the highest grades on the board exams, not only in the class but also in the entire nation. Collaborative, positive interactions are a blessing to all involved. What a contrast to the competitive atmosphere, which usually prevails.

Relationships and good fellowship are critical for each one of us and also very important in our community efforts. We need to be around people who love us and encourage us. We each seek compatible friends with whom we can be at ease. The effectiveness of our efforts to accomplish goals in life depends on the quality of our relationships with others and not how smart we are. This was clearly shown in our study of the TBL exercises with sophomore medical students.

CHAPTER 12

Contributions of Pharmacology to Society

Life's most persistent and urgent question is: What are you doing for others?

—Martin Luther King Jr.

Pharmacology is the study of the actions of drugs on living tissue. A pharmacologist tests the effects of drugs in animals with the hope of understanding mechanisms. My good friend Don Blake resigned his position as associate professor of pharmacology in the School of Pharmacy at Purdue. He was a good pharmacologist as well as a good Christian. He reasoned that if God can cure diseases by divine intervention, why do we need to bother testing drugs in animals? Isn't it simpler just to pray for these people? There are no bad side effects of prayer. Yes indeed, it is simpler to just pray, but for whatever reason, not everyone responds to prayer. Some people need a more substantive treatment. So pharmacology is an important area. Often the most tangible thing a physician can do for a patient is to write a prescription.

In 1957, I was a graduate student in pharmacology at Northwestern University Medical School and overheard a friendly debate between our faculties at the lunch table. One professor, Joseph "Jay" Wells, a fine, distinguished-looking man, made a point that drugs generally did not change the prognosis of diseases. Disease processes are strong and relentless, and drugs may relieve symptoms but do not alter the course of an illness. He admitted that there were a few exceptions, like anticoagulants and antibiotics, which had recently been developed, but most of the available drugs did not prolong life or substantially improve function. At that time, Dr. Wells was right, but now, we have many drugs that do, indeed, prolong life. This is especially true in the area of cardiovascular problems. The increase in longevity in the last several decades (in 1900, it was 47.3 years; in 1950, 68 years; and in 1998, 76.6 years) is due in part to the availability of new effective drugs, which can, indeed, change the course of a disease.

We have a fine deacon at our church who tells of being in a wheelchair twenty years ago due to severe arthritis in his knees. It was a very unpleasant experience, and he prayed that God would heal him. He went to the doctor who gave him an injection of a powerful new drug (Humira, a tumor necrosis factor blocker), and miraculously, the deacon was healed. He could walk again, praise the Lord! He thanks God for the miracle since God was the one who gave the pharmacologist the idea to make that new medication for arthritis. Thus, all healing comes from God, according to Deacon Jerry Cain. Some people may be healed directly by divine intervention, but others are healed through the ingenuity of men inspired by God.

When God heals directly, there are no side effects. When drugs are involved, side effects can occur. It's easy to take a pill or to have an injection, but that drug will generally permeate throughout the whole body, not only in the place it's needed. So drugs can be found in the saliva, tears, fingernails, and even in hair. Interestingly, someone analyzed a sample of Napoleon Bonaparte's hair and found high levels of the toxic metal arsenic and suggested that Napoleon may have died of arsenic poisoning. So both poisons and drugs can have a wide distribution in the body. Divine healing processes are similar to drugs in that they permeate all areas of the body, but they are a lot safer.

In 1964, I went to Winston Salem to teach pharmacology at the medical school associated with Wake Forest University. They had a technician there in pharmacology who had a wife and two little girls. When the wife was in her midtwenties, she was diagnosed with malignant hypertension. This is a severe form of the disease with rapidly escalating blood pressure and associated damage to blood vessels. Although her problem was accurately diagnosed, in those days (early 1950s), there were no good drugs for treatment of hypertension. There was nothing the doctors could do for her. She passed away about a year after diagnosis. The technician did not remarry but raised his daughters by himself. Many sad stories can be told about people dying young with high blood pressure. Hypertension is very common here in the USA, about 25 percent. In African Americans, it is even more common, 34 percent, practically an epidemic. It is called the "silent killer." People with hypertension feel great; there is no pain or discomfort. But there is progressive damage to blood vessels, and life span is shortened. When good antihypertensive drugs came out in the 1960s and 1970s, finally, physicians could prevent the early demise of these patients. The problem they have now is deciding which drug to use; there are so many good ones, beta-blockers, alpha-blockers, diuretics, calcium channel blockers, etc.

Hypertension is a complex disease and can be caused by a variety of factors. Two different patients may have identical pressures of 170 mm of mercury, but the cause of the hypertension may be different in the two patients. Drugs that work well in one of the patients may not work well in the other. We're blessed to have a variety of antihypertensives with different mechanisms so that we can take care of any type of high blood pressure. God makes provision for us all.

Atorvastatin (Lipitor) is the most popular of all drugs. This one single drug grossed $5.36 billion in 2009. It's popular and costs a lot, but it does a lot of good by blocking cholesterol synthesis mainly in the liver. Several studies show that when you lower blood cholesterol, you prolong life. Lipitor is the most popular of the statins, but several analogs are also used a lot. About 30 percent of the adults in the USA have high cholesterol. There is a great need for these lifesaving drugs.

We also have other drugs that can lower blood lipids by mechanisms different from the way statins work. For example, ezetimibe (Zetia) is often combined with a Lipitor-like drug because it blocks cholesterol absorption from the gut, which happens to be increased by Lipitor. These drugs work well together. Actually, there are six antilipid drug types among the top two hundred drugs on the market. Even if we don't exercise, eat properly, and take good care of ourselves, God still makes provision to help us.

Side effects are remarkably low with Lipitor-type drugs, thank God, but because so many people take them, a few have problems with muscle ache. When we move around, we damage skeletal muscle membranes and need to repair that damage using cholesterol, which is a constituent of cell membranes. Since Lipitor decreases cholesterol levels, less is available for muscle repair. If damage to membranes is severe, muscles can break down, releasing protein, which plugs up the kidneys in some people taking statins. Incidence of muscle problems is low in Lipitor patients especially if low doses are taken. So if you're taking statins in reasonable doses, muscle problems are unlikely. Please don't worry; trust God and your doctor.

Schizophrenia affects 1 percent of the population, and these people cannot function in society because of this disease. Many mental hospitals were constructed in the late 1800s and in the 1900s to accommodate schizophrenics. Then in the late 1950s, the drug chlorpromazine (Thorazine) appeared, and patients treated with this drug could be returned to their families and could function in society. Many mental institutions were closed because of the availability of chlorpromazine. It was a major advance and a great benefit to society since these patients were restored to the warmth and comfort of their own homes.

When I was a little boy in 1936, I went for a drive with my mom and dad in St. Louis, Missouri. Mom pointed out a building that was set back from the road and said it was a TB sanitarium where people with that disease were isolated from society and allowed to rest and, hopefully, recover their health. Every city had such places for these patients. Then in the 1960s, an effective antitubercular drug, isoniazid, was discovered, and TB sanitariums were no longer needed. TB patients were no longer infectious, could rejoin their families, and have a normal life.

Because of abortion and contraceptives, our world population is only half of what it would be otherwise. The combination oral contraceptives, which contain both estrogen and progestin, block ovulation. They do away with the menstrual cycle so there is no possibility of conception.

However, the progestin-only pill blocks ovulation only 75 percent of the time, so conception can still take place in 25 percent of the women. Thus, in 2.5 percent of the women fertilized, ova implant as normally in the uterine wall and pregnancy occurs despite the use of the progestin-only contraceptive. However, implantation sometimes occurs in the fallopian tube since progestin inhibits movement of the egg toward the uterus. Tubal pregnancies are not sustainable and must be terminated. Lastly, progestin can alter the uterine lining so the egg cannot implant. Then the fertilized ovum passes out with the urine and is lost. Many believe that the fertilized ovum is a human being, and therefore, the use of progestin-only oral contraceptives is considered unethical by pro-life physicians.

In the mid-1990s, AIDS (human immunodeficiency virus infection) was a fatal disease. If you contracted AIDS, it was a death sentence, and you were bound to die in a few years. There was no cure. The prognosis was grim. Then in 1997, a new antiretroviral drug, Crixivan, came out, and if this drug is taken each day, AIDS is not fatal, but it's just a chronic problem. Now, AIDS patients can live a normal life span by taking Crixivan. Man's God-given ingenuity can bring about miracles.

Pharmacology has had a great, beneficial impact on our society by promoting health, prolonging many lives, restoring family situations by eliminating the need to isolate patients from the rest of society, and by giving us all the security of knowing that if we're not well, drugs can help.

CHAPTER 13

A Commentary on Modern Medical Practice

Where there is great love, there are always miracles.

—Willa Cather

Issam Nemeh is in his fifties, an MD from Syria, and a devout Christian. He was trained in surgery and anesthesiology but switched to acupuncture to enable him to interact more with patients. He has an enormously successful practice in Cleveland, Ohio. He has a deep faith in the healing power of the Holy Spirit and often is able to discern both what the patient's problem is and the prognosis. Not only is he a good physician, but he also has godly insight into medical situations (*Miracles Every Day*, Maura Poston Zagrans, Doubleday Religion, 2010).

Maura Zagrans shares a personal story about Dr. Nemeh's wife. She asked the doctor one night who he was. She had been married to him twenty-five years, and he was still an enigma to her. He left the room and brought back a picture of a painting of Christ's entry into Jerusalem on Palm Sunday. He answered her question with another question. Who in the painting would you like to be? He then commented that he was trying to be the one closest to Christ. He was trying to be the donkey. His humility and desire to serve are well illustrated by this story.

Issam works long hours usually from 9:00 a.m. to midnight, six days a week. He takes as much time as necessary for each patient and often adds prayer to his treatment regimen. He has seen miraculous healings for cancer and other serious problems. People from all over seek his help, and it takes months to get an appointment with him. You may think that this is a strange man, but he has a relatively normal life with a wife and four children. Actually, his wife is his office manager, and there is an interesting story behind their relationship.

Both Dr. Nemeh and his wife are from Syria. She was being courted by a tall, handsome medical student in that country. The custom there is for the potential groom to have a party with both his family and the potential bride's family. At the appropriate time, the young man proposes a toast in the presence of the two families and asks the young lady to marry him. When the time came for the toast, the glass shattered in the young man's hand, and the proposal was never made. Soon after this event, Issam began seeing Kathy, and eventually, they were married. It seems as though this woman were divinely chosen for him so that Dr. Nemeh's medical practice could flourish and many people would benefit.

Dr. Nemeh spends six days a week in a three-room office suite about a mile from his home. Once there, he doesn't leave, and Kathy cooks lunch and dinner for Issam and his two secretaries and any volunteers who happen to be there. Furnishings are modest but adequate. Cookies, candy, and pretzels are available for patients and families, and they feel very much at ease in the waiting room. Patients are charged for acupuncture since medical insurance companies don't pay for this service.

Some healings are instantaneous. A woman, who was a physical therapist herself, sustained neck, thigh, and shoulder injuries in a bicycle accident. Despite intensive therapy for a year, she had only a thirty-degree range of motion in one arm. She was discouraged and thought she might not ever be healed. She went to Dr. Nemeh, and the doctor examined her and got up from his wheeled chair and stood behind her. He announced that she was going to be healed and told her to raise her arms and move them back and forth. In a few minutes, the range of movement improved, and function was restored to normal. She was so elated that she went to her parents' home and shared the good news with them. Years later, she described her healing, "No more specialists! No more physical, ortho-, neuro-, and massotherapy! I became fully functional and could do everything without pain and without restriction." Thank God for talented physicians like Dr. Nemeh.

A man who was president of a computer service company went to repair a family computer. While he was working on the computer, he complained to the customer of neck pain. He had been to a chiropractor and sustained a ruptured disk during therapy. He was awaiting surgery and was in great discomfort. The customer referred him to Dr. Nemeh. He took his MRIs showing the ruptured disk with him. During acupuncture therapy, Dr. Nemeh prayed for the patient and after ten minutes asked him how he felt. The patient opened his mouth to reply and heard a snap in the back of his neck. The pain was gone. Both men knew what happened, and the patient thanked Dr. Nemeh and started to get up from the chair. Dr. Nemeh asked where he was going and told him he was not done with him yet and that he still had no feeling in the fingers on his right hand. The patient had not mentioned this problem, so there was no obvious way for the doctor to have known about it. So therapy continued till the patient was completely healed. Another "Holy Bingo" allowed cancellation of the planned surgery.

Issam Nemeh's parents recall that he was a very unusual infant. He never cried or fussed but was self-content. As a child, he spent much time at a local church, praying or talking to a priest. On the playground, he would pray for those who fell or were hurt. He knew a religious theme would dominate his life. "The word *religion* comes from the Latin *religare*, or retying, thus religion is the science of reconnecting souls to their Creator." This was Dr. Nemeh's destiny.

Zagrans, in her book on Dr. Nemeh, explains that prayer stimulates the anterior cingulate gyrus of the brain, where a balance between thought and feeling occurs and decreases activity in the limbic system, where strong emotions like anger are expressed. Prayer thus enhances empathy and compassion and overrides destructive and less rational actions of the hippocampus, amygdala, fornix, and other limbic structures.

Issam Nemeh insists there is nothing special about him. He resents being called a faith healer. He says, "God and God alone heals." This is a fact that every physician should be aware of. No matter how clever the therapy devised by the physician, healing comes from the Almighty One. Dr. Nemeh says his only gift is one of faith, the assurance that when he approaches a patient, he knows that God can and will deliver a healing. We are the ones who put limitations on God.

One patient's husband asked Dr. Nemeh, "How can you sit in this office from early morning till God knows when, day after day? How do you do it?" This is a poignant question considering the mix of profound illness and related desperation involved in Dr. Nemeh's practice. Time is irrelevant, said Dr. Nemeh. The dedication of this man is amazing and supernatural. He says he is honored to devote himself to God, and it is the Holy Spirit who sustains him.

Some healings are not so sudden. One woman was diagnosed with stage 4 non-Hodgkin's lymphoma. She went into remission after eight months of chemotherapy but broke her leg a year later, and it calcified, abnormally leaving her with a marked limp. She went to Dr. Nemeh, and after two hours' treatment, her foot straightened but not completely. However, she was now able to walk up steps and do some gardening without pain. Over a period of two years, further acupuncture treatments brought about a complete healing. She said when Dr. Nemeh concentrates on helping others, he loses his own agenda. This reflects Issam's great ability to focus on his God-given task.

Dr. Nemeh met a Catholic nun who invited him to a prayer service in the nearby convent. Afterward, the nun would drop by Dr. Nemeh's office for social visits periodically. On one occasion, the nun felt compelled to visit, and Issam felt compelled to ask her to stay for treatment. The woman waiting for the next appointment gave up her turn to allow Dr. Nemeh to treat the nun. Kathy thanked the lady and said it was very nice of her since you never know how long the doctor will spend with a patient. "There you are with a terrible pain in your knee and you gave your time to Sister, God bless you."

During the time Dr. Nemeh spent with the nun, the lady remained in the waiting room, and her knee became very warm. After it stopped pulsating, the pain was gone. Apparently, some of Dr. Nemeh's patients are cured in the waiting room even before they see Issam. Kathy told her it happened because she was so generous in giving up her appointment time and that she could go home.

Upon examining the nun, Dr. Nemeh discovered a tumor in a salivary gland (parotid) that needed immediate attention by an ear, nose, and throat (ENT) specialist. The adenocarcinoma was largely entwined around the facial nerve, making surgery difficult with many possible complications. So the nun went to the ENT specialist who had a sign in his office, "We treat; Jesus heals." She knew she was in the right place. Dr. Nemeh gave the nun acupuncture therapy at 2:00 a.m. on the day of her scheduled surgery, and she felt something pop in her neck. Later, during surgery, the doctor found the tumor had regressed and was no longer entwined around the facial nerve. It was removed with minimum complications. Then, miraculously, they found the tumor was not malignant after all, and chemotherapy was not necessary. How intricate are these important events in the process of godly healing.

Not everyone who goes to Dr. Nemeh is healed. One lady went to him with serious cancer. By looking at her, he knew that God was calling her home. He counseled her, and she died peacefully two weeks later. We all have to die, and it was time for this lady to go home. The insight of Dr. Nemeh is incredible, and the ability to lead this lady gently from this life into the next is a great miracle in itself.

Dr. Nemeh has a novel approach to the practice of medicine. He is in no hurry with the patient; he takes his time to get to know the individual and carefully plans his treatment strategy. He sometimes asks the patient to cancel a scheduled surgery, and complete healing takes place. We need more physicians like Issam. This man is unusually successful, and other physicians would do well to conduct their business accordingly. Yes, we need specialists, but for the average patient, people like Dr. Nemeh are what are needed in abundance. Some patients must wait almost a year to get to see Issam. Perhaps medical education should make provision for people who have Dr. Nemeh's ability, maybe by having an elective course in the third year.

CHAPTER 14

Divine Healing versus Modern Medicine

The toughest thing about being a success is that you've got to keep being a success.

—Irving Berlin

If divine healing is so good and so powerful with no side effects, why are there so many people in hospitals? If you are a deep believer in Holy Scripture, you know that Christ healed all who came to Him. We previously quoted Matthew 9:35, which says, "Jesus went about . . . healing every sickness and every disease among the people." He didn't turn anybody away. He never said, "I'm sorry, your condition is too serious for me, you'll have to see someone else." He healed everyone. Why isn't divine healing more common at the present time?

Has the power of the Holy Spirit dissipated over the centuries? No, since some instances of divine healing still occur. It seems to me that God is still the all-powerful creator and is eternal. He has not changed, and his power is undiminished and still available today for those who believe. Romans 8:11 says, "But if the Spirit of him who raised Christ from the dead dwells in you, he who raised Christ from the dead will also give life to your mortal bodies through his Spirit who dwells in you."

Furthermore, in Matthew 13:15, Christ says, "The hearts of this people have grown dull, their ears are hard of hearing, and their eyes they have closed, lest they should see with their eyes and hear with their ears, lest they should understand with their hearts and in turn so that I should heal them." Doubt and unbelief on the part of the patient or their relatives or friends or attending medical personnel is harmful and can interfere with the healing process.

The society we live in today is science oriented. We believe in science but doubt everything else. We are like the people of Nazareth in the time of Christ in our unbelief. This may explain why divine healing is less common today.

I spoke to my pastor, Father David Buckles about the scarcity of divine healing nowadays. He answered that it still occurs commonly, but they attribute it to drugs and doctors now. I can see the truth in his comment and am grateful to him for his wisdom.

I went to a Full Gospel meeting at which the speaker talked about his healing from acute appendicitis. Foolish as it may seem, he was convinced that he didn't need to go to a doctor for his appendicitis. His wife was in full agreement and completely supported him. She carefully screened all visitors and allowed only those who were positive and supportive to visit, believing that a doubtful attitude can interfere with healing. The man was completely healed of his appendicitis. We can have a great physical influence on one another according to the depth of our spirituality.

Joel Osteen, the famous pastor and TV evangelist, tells the story of his grandmother. She had serious liver cancer years ago when chemotherapy and radiotherapy were not very effective treatments. She decided not to have any therapy at all and to pray for divine healing. She lost a lot of weight and looked bad, but she continued to have a positive attitude. Her family understood and was also positive and encouraging. Slowly, she overcame the problem and lived for twenty-five years. Hers was an amazing story of God's power to heal.

I visited a man in the hospital who was unconscious and dying of leukemia. He couldn't eat, and his kidney and gastrointestinal functions were failing. His wife was there, and there was a golf tournament on TV. It was summer outside, but the atmosphere in the room contrasted with the golf and the summer weather. I tried to say something positive, so I mentioned that you never know what the Holy Spirit will do. He may come into Gary's body, and he may get up and go outside and run around the block. A couple of minutes later, he woke up. A mere mention of something positive apparently was enough to rouse that man from a coma. I didn't have enough sense to pray out loud for the man's healing, but he was well enough to have a brief conversation with his wife. It seemed to me that there was a negative pall over the room, which would have been difficult to overcome. For the Holy Spirit to work his healing miracles, deep belief without doubt or negativity is needed.

CHAPTER 15

Importance of Relationships

Love cures all people—both the ones who give it and the ones who receive it.

—Dr. Karl Menninger

Love is a strong potion. It permeates every cell of your body, bringing peace, joy, and health. How good it is to know someone loves you despite your failures, warts and all. It carries healing in its wings and counteracts any negativity or any burdens you might have. The powerful medicinal effect of God's love and the strong, unconditional love of other human beings is a great blessing, and all the love you have needs to be cherished as your most precious possession.

Ron Rolheiser is a famous theologian who is currently president of the Oblate School of Theology in San Antonio, Texas. In an interview published in the *St. Anthony Messenger,* March 2013, he mentions an essay entitled "In Praise of Skin" by Brenda Peterson. She had a skin rash and tried every doctor and every ointment she could buy. They even gave her cortisone shots, but nothing worked. Then her grandmother, who was a midwife, said, "You know what's wrong with you? The skin has to be touched." Her grandmother then began massage therapy for her, and the skin rash went away. That loving, wholesome physical contact is so important to each of us, makes us feel loved and accepted, and can bring about a profound healing. This may explain the existence of massage parlors. We are not happy living in isolation.

After many good years of teaching, including awards for excellence, Dr. Willis Tacker, MD, PhD, retired from our medical faculty at Purdue last year. He gave a short talk to the students and faculty at our annual spring dinner. He quoted from the Shakespearean play, *The Tempest*. The original quote was by the character Prospero. Dr. Tacker modified the quote and said to the students, "You are the stuff of my dreams." He was saying it was a privilege for him to contribute to the careers of these fine young people who will positively influence many lives in our society. It made him feel good to participate in such a worthwhile program. This heartfelt sentiment was very much appreciated by the students. I believe all our medical faculty have the same feelings about the work we do. We can say as Dr. Tacker says, "I have the best job in the world."

Sometimes, however, there is understandable tension between medical students and faculty. Students have a need and strong desire to know the material. They all want to be outstanding physicians and competent in their work. If the faculty member doesn't describe the importance of the subject efficiently and make clear and interesting points, the students get upset. I know one faculty member who used to sweat profusely during his lectures. His shirt would be soaked with sweat after he taught a class. I didn't always do well either; some years were better than others.

Sometimes, I get too animated and overly enthusiastic, and it becomes comic. I have had students laugh out loud at me. It was a great embarrassment. But then I thought, they were justified, and it told me something about my lecture style. Since then, I have tried to be more urbane and less animated.

I used to think up questions to ask the students during my lectures. Things that I thought they should know and pertinent to the lecture, like what is the cardiac output and how much does it increase during exercise. Usually, one of the students would come up with the right answer. But it really added nothing to the lecture and taught them nothing new. Also, it put them ill at ease. They had to be on their guard and be ready to answer questions. They were not in a receptive, learning mode. Eliminating these questions greatly improved the class.

Medical problems are not the most joyful things to talk about. Pathology, all kinds of diseases, drug side effects, etc., can be depressing topics. So I try to have some jokes to tell for each lecture. These are told about twenty minutes after beginning the lecture when student's minds usually begin to wander. I try to have as many medical jokes as possible. Like the one about the lady who was driving to the grocery store with her little four-year-old daughter in the backseat. The lady was a physician and had left her stethoscope there in the backseat. She looked in the rearview mirror and noticed her daughter was playing with the stethoscope. She was thrilled thinking that maybe her daughter would follow in her footsteps and become a physician. Just then the little girl put the instrument up to her mouth and said, "Welcome to McDonald's." Many of the jokes are corny, but anything to bring some joy and improve relationships is useful.

Once I embarrassed myself talking to one student whose name was Brenton Goodman. He was a very good and competent student. I was trying to compliment him and told him he was a good man. I then realized what I had done, and it was an awkward moment. He was nice about it and just smiled.

One thing I learned early on is that I cannot go to a social function the night before a lecture. I must concentrate on the material and get a good night's sleep. Also, I skip breakfast when I lecture in the morning. Fasting clears my head and relaxes me. Fasting and prayer are known to be powerful weapons in spiritual warfare. Relationships, basically, are spiritual challenges, and biblical principles apply here. It's critically important that I have a godly, loving attitude toward each and every student in the class. Otherwise, I cannot be an effective teacher.

One year, I got a really bad teaching evaluation from the medical students. Somehow, I turned them off early in the fall, and it made for a long, frustrating year. They met with me to express their concerns. They said I needed to highlight the important points in the handouts and that they could not remember everything I said, so I needed to slow down. I tried to adjust to their criticisms, but apparently, it wasn't enough. I thank God that I felt little animosity toward them and was able to finish the year without losing my composure. It took a lot of prayer and fasting to accomplish this. Teaching medical students is God's business, and he gives strength to those who call upon him. Isaiah 41:10 says, "Fear not, I am with you, do not be dismayed, I am your God, I will strengthen you and help you, I will uphold you with my victorious right hand."

Even so, I felt bad about the situation and talked it over with the dean. I thought I might be fired. Thank God, the dean, Dr. Gordon Coppoc, is a fine Christian man, and he understood since something similar had happened to him a few years before. He suggested I look carefully at the lectures and revise them as best I could. I did so, but still I had a lot of anxiety the whole next year. Thank God that year's class was an exceptionally good one, and it went OK.

As a medical faculty member, one of the greatest joys is to witness a young person immersed in all the scientific details of our program also develop a deep appreciation of the spiritual aspects of medicine. Justin Colanese played golf along with Ben Petty, Alex Serafin, and me after the pharmacology course was over. He was not only an excellent golfer but he was also intelligent and competent. At our spring dinner, he mentioned how much he appreciated the efforts of Dr. Charlie Babbs, one of our outstanding faculty members, for his enthusiastic teaching. Despite all his good qualities, something was missing in Justin's life. He did not have the equanimity of William Osler, nor did he appreciate the spiritual aspects of medicine.

Justin was dating a girl he was serious about. She broke off the relationship with him because he wasn't a Christian. He was deeply hurt, but as he thought about it, he realized the girl was right. Something important was missing in his life. When Justin became a Christian during his final years of medical school, he blossomed into a well-rounded, capable medical student.

Another student in the same class, Julie Stark, was a fine Christian woman who won the Gold Humanism Award that year. This award is given to students who show great empathy and consideration for others. I remember I was trying to make a point in class but was interrupted by a question. In answering the question, I forgot what point I was going to make. Julie was kind enough and insightful enough to remind me of what was being discussed and saved the moment. I deeply appreciated what she did.

Two medical students, Josh Tierney and Matt Hoskins, are among the finest human beings I've ever known. Josh Tierney came by to visit me in the hospital. Busy as he was, he took the time to come to see me. I really appreciated his thoughtfulness. We discussed his desire to become a medical missionary several times when he took pharmacology. He has a good heart and a deep commitment to serve those in need. My friend, Joann Clark and I attended his wedding in an old church in Indianapolis. It was the most beautiful wedding Joann and I ever witnessed. A small combo played, and the ceremony was relatively informal. The pastor knew both of them well and performed a very intimate ceremony. The bride was not feeling good, but it worked out well anyway. Josh was very attentive to her, and he made a profound impression with his statement that he would always love her even if she hurt his feelings.

Joann and I had purchased a large cooking pot about fifteen inches in diameter and about fifteen inches deep as a wedding gift. It was very expensive, but it was on their gift list. We thought they might want it for use in a soup kitchen. Apparently, it was a mistake, and it was not on their gift list after all, but they were able to return it. We had a good laugh about it.

Matt Hoskins was a top student in his medical class and a very gracious man. He was the main speaker for his class at his first spring dinner and did an excellent job of relating to both faculty and students present there. He has outstanding leadership abilities. His father, also, is a physician, and they went to Pakistan together on a medical mission before his sophomore year. I met both his father and his mother and was impressed with the fact that they are such a fine Christian family.

Toward the end of his stay at Lafayette Center for Medical Education (LCME), Matt Hoskins arranged for a missionary physician to Gabon, Africa, to speak to our medical students and faculty. Since it was late on a Thursday night, a catered meal was provided. Matt served as host. He made us all feel welcome and had the courage to say a blessing before the meal and to thank God for all he does for us. This occurred at Purdue, a secular institution, and warmed the hearts of all the well-meaning, godly people present, students and faculty alike.

On one exam over a series of difficult lectures covering a lot of details, Matt aced the exam. I couldn't believe it. No one had ever done that before. The powerful combination of intellect and deep spirituality in Matt is truly amazing. I'm grateful to God for calling such a fine young man like Matt into the medical profession.

Josh and Matt are just two examples of the high quality of people in the medical classes. These students are outstanding individuals, and I believe they are destined to do many good things in their medical careers. Just being in their presence makes you feel good. Love for mankind radiates from them. God does indeed pick special people to serve human beings, the greatest of his creation, in the capacity of physicians.

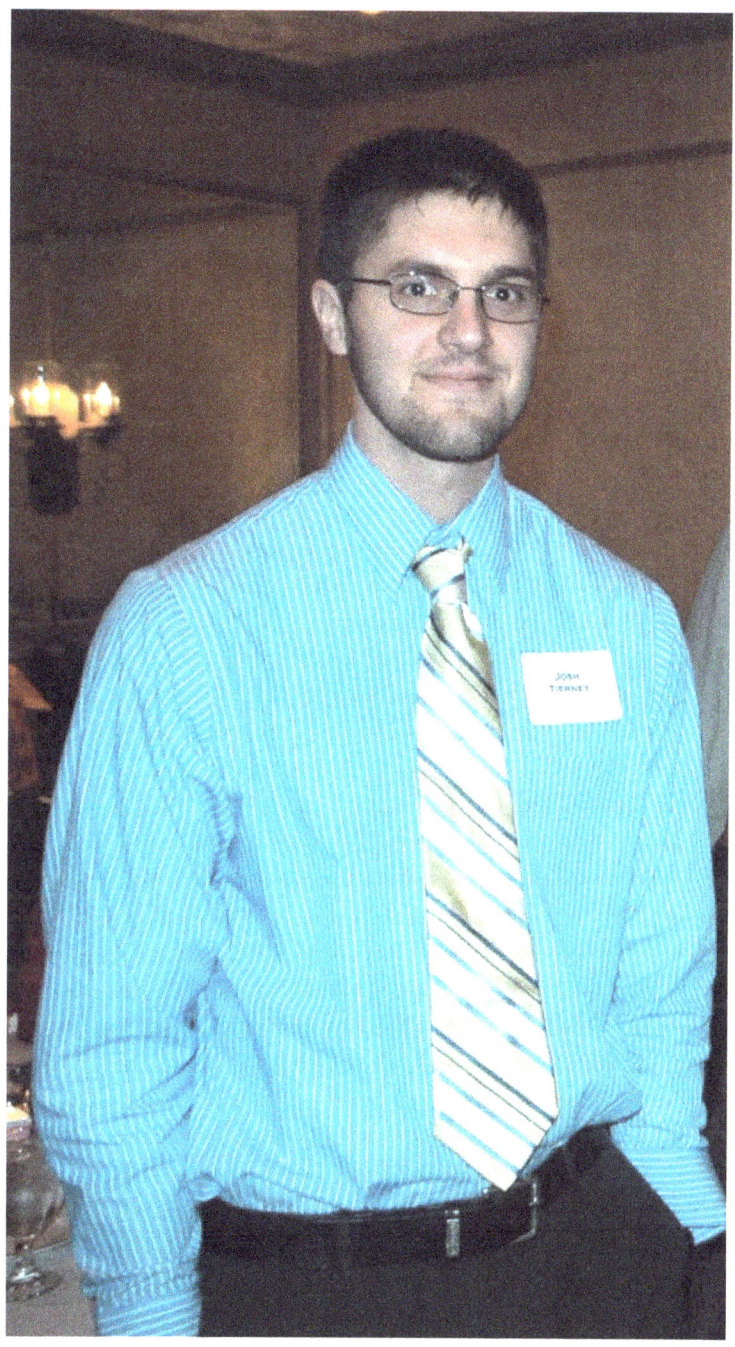

This is Josh Tierney at the Spring Dinner in 2005; an outstanding medical student and a fine Christian man intent on doing missionary work. No doubt that this man will be a fine surgeon and be of great benefit and an inspiration to many people in his career.

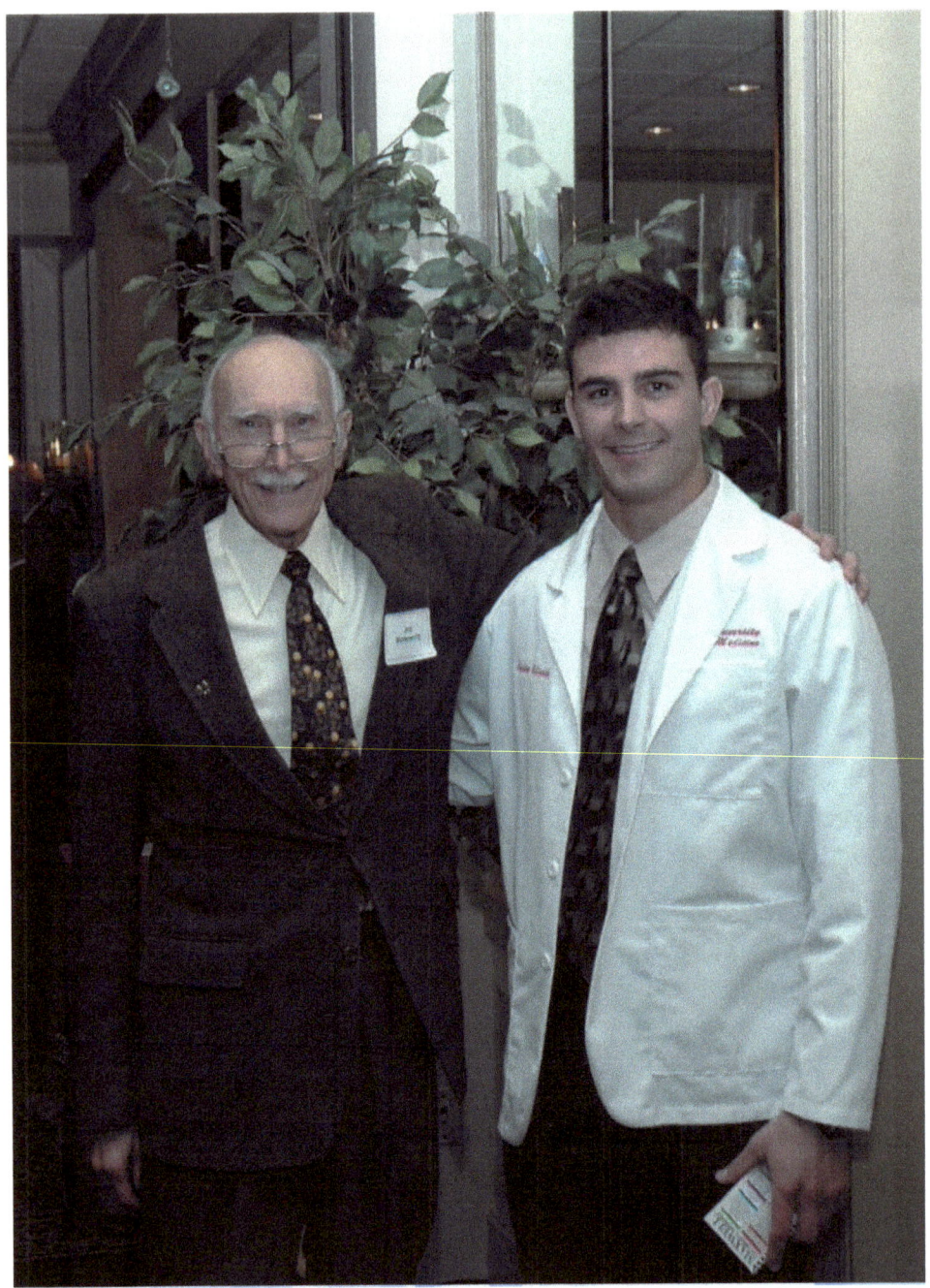

This is Justin Colanese at the Spring Dinner in 2009. At this time he was a very good medical student and a pleasant young man. But later he had a deep experience with the Holy Spirit and a radical improvement occurred. When the Holy Spirit enters your heart, you rise above your earthly capabilities and joy in abundance pours forth.

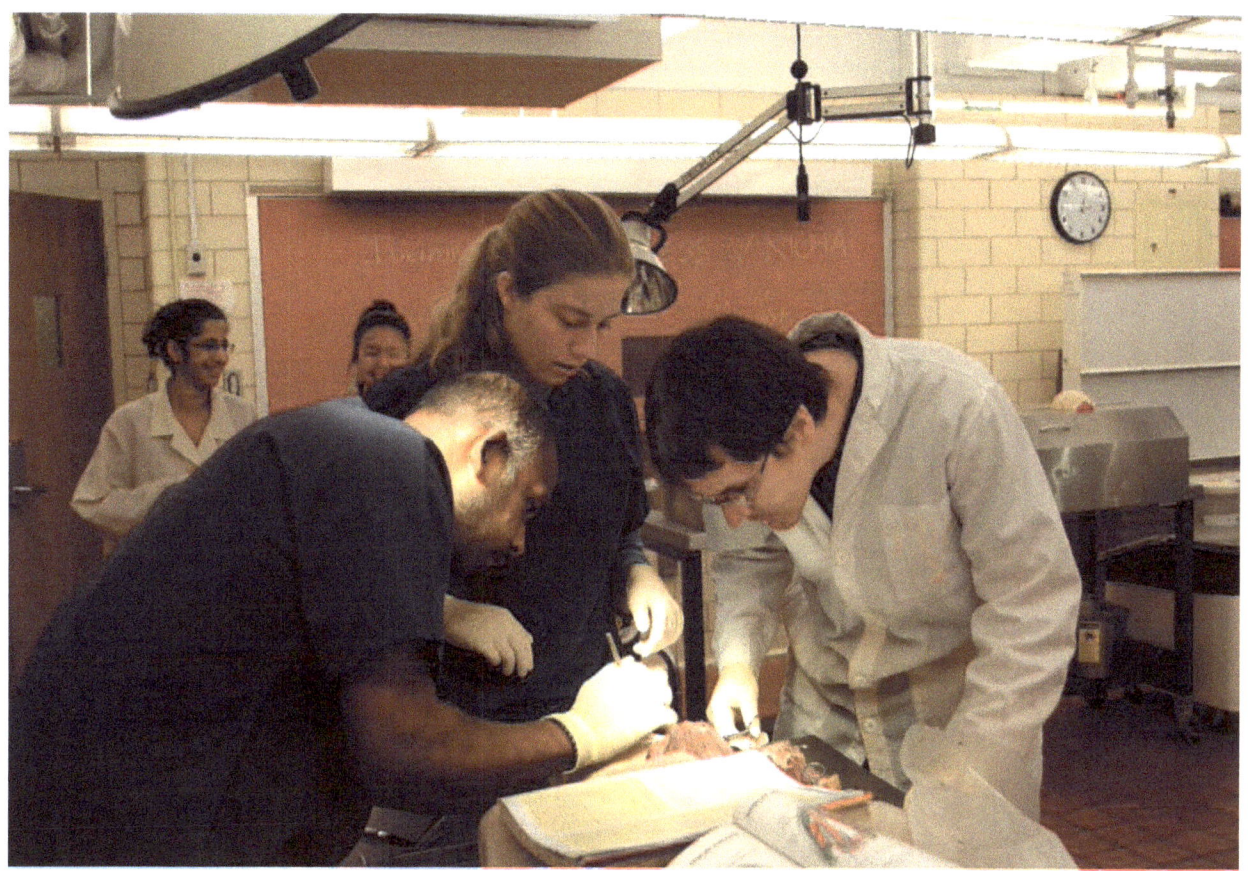

Matt Hoskins on the right in anatomy lab with Mary Ann Cladis and Velu Balasubramanian. All three were brilliant students but Matt was one of the finest people I have ever known. His father is also a physician. I've met his mother too and she, like the rest of the family, is a fine Christian lady.

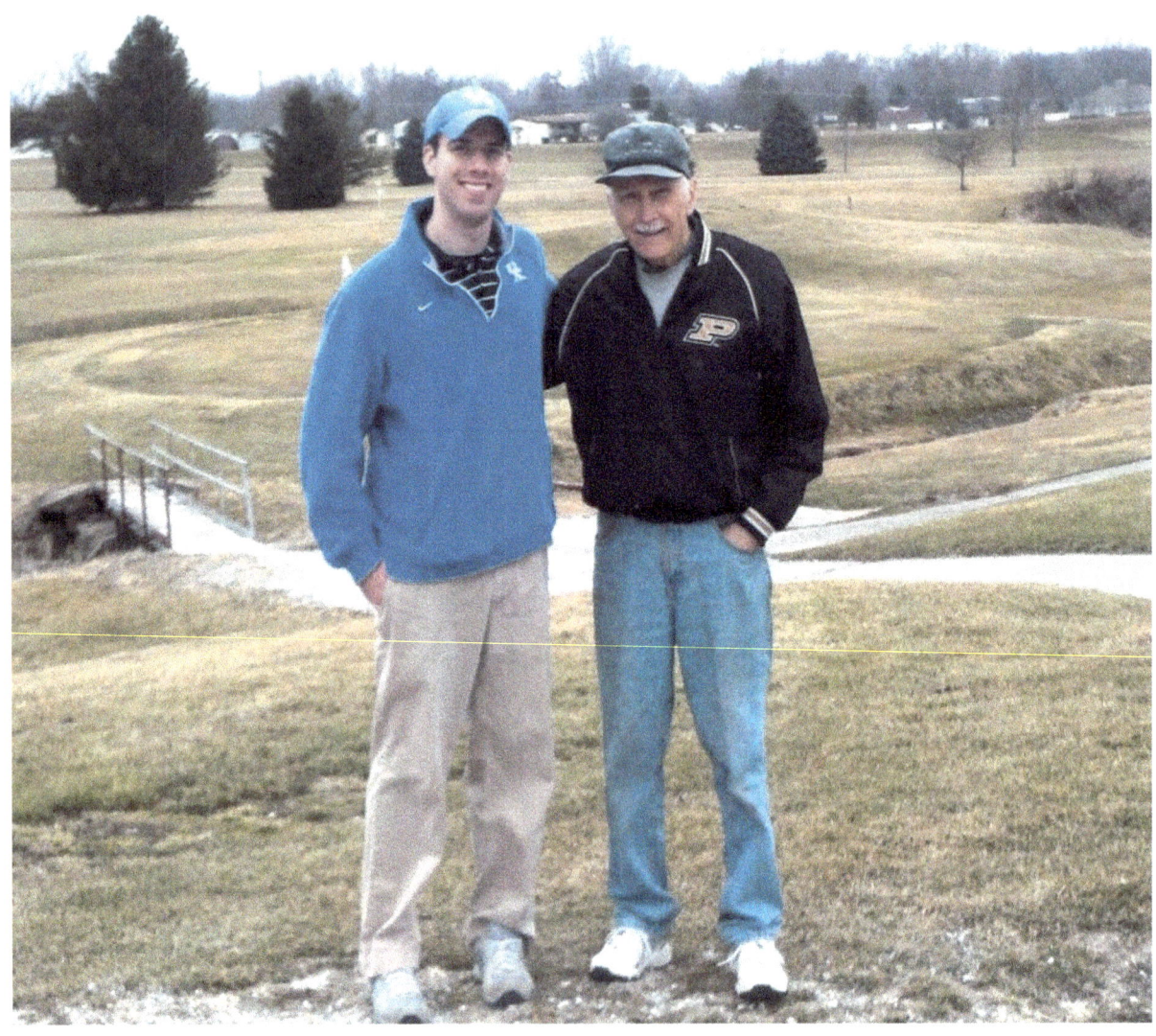

In March of 2013 after I had finished my pharmacology lectures, Cody Bearden, Drew Schmidt and I played golf at Edwood Glen Country Club in West Lafayette, IN. It was cloudy and cool but not bad for March and we had a good time. Both are strong young men and hit the ball a long way. Cody had to leave early to meet his wife so he is not in the photo.

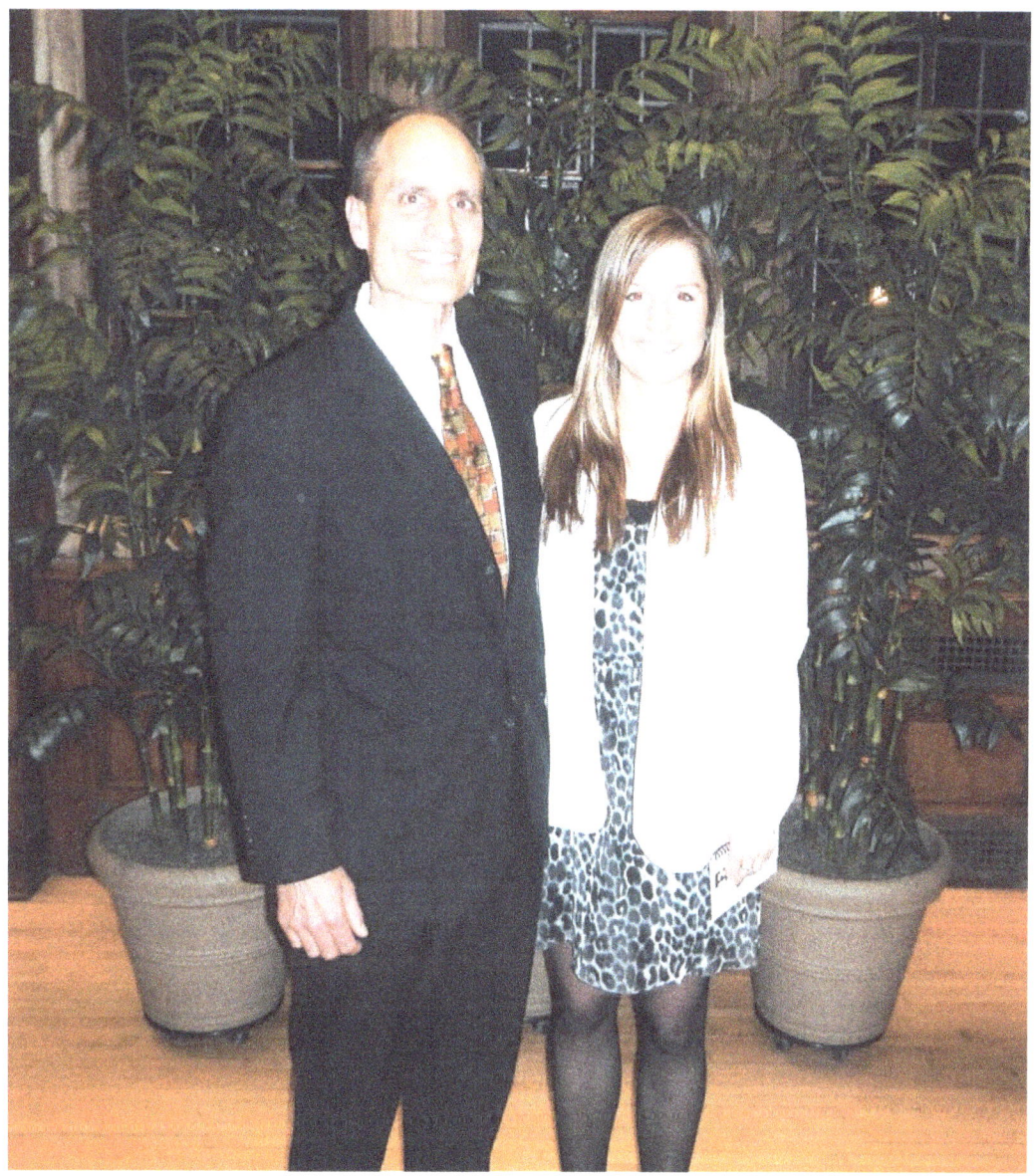

This is Mary Rush and her father Jim at the Spring Dinner for medical students in 2013. Her mother is a Supreme Court Judge for the State of Indiana and her father is a Deacon in the Catholic Church. Mary is also an outstanding person and has a reputation for being one of the most compassionate individuals we ever had in our program. Obviously this is a very important characteristic for a physician to have. She will be a valuable help to her patients using both a deep spiritual and an insightful scientific approach.

CHAPTER 16

Conclusion

I know the plans I have for you, says the Lord, plans for welfare and not for evil, to give you a future and a hope.

—Jeremiah 29:11

An important point of this book is to offer some possible explanations for why a godly lifestyle is associated with health and longevity. Why do churchgoers live longer than others? Maybe because of good personal interactions with other people, no alcohol or cigarettes, healthy lifestyle, godly habits, etc. Maybe there are several reasons, but probably, the most important is that these people are closer to God. He's the one who determines our destiny. He naturally gives life and takes it away.

Individual examples don't allow for statistics, but I'd like to mention a couple of people who support the idea that a godly lifestyle leads not only to longevity but also to fullness of life.

A good friend of mine was a librarian, a sweet little old lady with varicose veins, Bernice Cloutier. She was a gentle, likeable person who never married. She died about five years ago at the age of one hundred. Always a quiet, soft-spoken, slow-moving, thin woman, but she was very active in the Charismatic movement. She went to the Full Gospel Meetings and Charismatic Conferences at Notre Dame University and enjoyed them enormously. When she spoke at our local Charismatic meetings, it was always very powerful. She spoke of Jesus as her boyfriend with whom she was going steady. It was a wild, fantastic love affair, and she was ecstatically happy about it. I visited her once when she was in a nursing home. She had a little vertigo (dizziness). She couldn't understand how her boyfriend could allow her to be so afflicted, but she knew everything was going to be OK. So life was not always a bed of roses for her either, but she always had a positive hope and trusted in God's love for her.

Another good friend of mine was Sister Frances Mary, a nun of the Precious Blood Order. I took my daughter to see her on Halloween one year. My daughter was about five years old, and we got her a tiger suit with a long tiger tail that stuck straight out behind her. It was a riot. Sister and the other nuns were overjoyed to see her walk around their living room with her long tiger tail trailing behind. I visited Sister Francis Mary when she was deathly ill in hospice. She was weak and, obviously, not feeling good, yet there she was praising God for the life he had given her. She lived in a convent house on East State Street in Lafayette, Indiana, with about ten other nuns. They made communion bread for the local Catholic churches. She died in her nineties. It was a servile existence, but she was so grateful for the life God had given her, you would have thought she was a queen. However, with a loving congregation of nuns and the many friends who cherished her, life for her was a joyful experience.

I'm reminded of all the times I went to see a doctor and really didn't need to do so. As a young man, I sprained my ankle playing basketball. It swelled up and was a problem to me. The doctor laughed when he saw me. There was really nothing he could do to help. God already made plans for healing the ankle. It was only a matter of time. Also, I played football in the eighth grade, a ninety-pound right halfback. I got cleated twice in the inner aspect of the left ankle. Football cleats are dull and don't break the skin but leave a deep bruise. When I was in college, I went to see a doctor because of the slight swelling beneath the skin in the bruised ankle area. I thought it might be a tumor. He said it was a buildup of scar tissue and nothing to worry about.

Working for a PhD at Northwestern and under a lot of stress, I got the idea that I had multiple sclerosis (MS), a chronic neurodegenerative disease. I remember calling my mother and telling her. I read in *Merck Manual* (usually a reliable medical text describing disease) that scintillating scotoma (jagged, colored, flashing lights) was pathognomonic (sure sign of a disease) for MS. I was terribly upset about my scintillating scotoma and at the prospect of becoming an invalid. I had trouble concentrating on my work. I talked to Dr. North, my PhD adviser, about it. He was doing a residency in anesthesiology and knew the physicians at Wesley Memorial Hospital across the street. He made an appointment for me to see Dr. Paul Bucy, a famous neurologist for whom the Klüver-Bucy syndrome was named. Dr. Bucy examined me and told me that he himself sometimes saw jagged, colored, flashing lights, so he too had scintillating scotoma and that it was not pathognomonic for MS. Dr. Bucy and Dr. North probably had a good laugh about me. But I'm embarrassed to say that I didn't believe Dr. Bucy. I still worried for several years thinking I had MS. How important it is to have faith in a loving, healing God. We take reasonably good care of our health, but mainly, it's God's business, and we just need to concentrate on building his kingdom on earth.

In the USA, at the present time, we do not have a balanced approach to medical treatment. (Dr. Nemeh is an exception.) There is too much emphasis on evidence-based therapy. I'm told that many foreign countries have a more coordinated approach. In this country, people in the medical professions as well as the general public need to understand the importance of both the scientific and spiritual aspects of disease.

There needs to be a dual scientific/spiritual attack on health problems. Let me share an important true story with you. Oral Roberts University (ORU) Medical School in Tulsa, Oklahoma, had a strong science-based and Charismatic Christian curriculum, but it had to be closed in 1989 due to financial problems. The students then involved in the ORU program were bona fide, high-quality students and needed to be transferred to another medical school. After some difficulty, another medical school was found to take on the ORU students. However, some problems arose when the patients in the university hospital much preferred the ORU students with their deeply spiritual orientation, and not the host university students despite their strong science background. This story was told to me by faculty from Harvard Medical School who knew the situation created by closing of the ORU Medical Program. It emphasizes the need of a strong spiritual approach to medical training and practice.

So what's the answer for the question "Is disease mainly a scientific or a spiritual problem"? Obviously, it's both, and God shows us how to handle it scientifically and spiritually. To me, the spiritual aspects are more important than the scientific.

Jesus said, "I have come that you may have life and life in all its fullness" (John 10:10). Never before was I so happy as when I was baptized in the Holy Spirit, and that joy has continued through the following thirty-eight years. Despite many trials and tribulations, it remains as a pinnacle experience for me and marks a point in my life where an important change for the better occurred. A strong desire to follow the guidance of the Holy Spirit and to serve the Lord with all your heart makes life worthwhile.

INDEX

A

acupuncture, 104, 106
Adams, Patch, 89

B

Blake, Don, 42, 97
Borch, Rick, 70-71
Bucy, Paul, 130

C

Catholic Church, 35, 44, 126
Chaplain Hinson, 90-91
Charismatic movement, 35, 44-45, 57, 128
cholesterol, 101
Christian Pharmacy Student Association, 14, 57, 64
Christian Pharmacy Student Group, 61-62
Colanese, Justin, 118-19, 123
contraceptives, 102
Cousins, Norman, 86-88

D

divine healing, 45, 48, 50, 53, 59-60, 78, 111-13
drugs, 18, 26-27, 30, 32, 71, 80, 82, 97-101, 103, 112

F

Father Martin, 91
Fredrichs, Edward, 83-85
Full Gospel Business Men, 42, 44

G

Gibson, Leslie, 88-89
God, 9, 11-16, 21, 28, 32-35, 42-43, 45-47, 49, 51-52, 55-58, 60-62, 69, 71, 75, 81, 85, 90-92, 97-98, 100-101, 106-8, 110-11, 113-14, 117-18, 120-21, 127-31

H

healing, 9, 14-15, 45, 48-52, 59-60, 79, 86, 89, 98, 106, 108, 111-15, 129
Hinson, Jack, 90-91
Holy Spirit, 43-46, 49-51, 65-69, 72-73, 75, 85, 104, 108, 111, 113, 123, 131
Hoskins, Matt, 119-21, 124
hypertension, 99-100

J

Jesus Christ, 21, 42, 46, 48-49, 53, 56, 58, 62, 73, 105, 111-12, 128, 131

K

Koenig, Harold, 75

L

Lafayette Center for Medical Education (LCME), 38, 72, 78, 120
Lamborene, 81-82, 89
laughter, 87-93
Lipitor, 100-101
love, 13, 35, 54, 58, 73-75, 79, 85, 96, 114, 119, 121, 128

M

Maickel, Roger, 70-71
miracles, 9, 15-16, 34, 50, 56, 66, 79, 98, 103-4
MS (multiple sclerosis), 129-30

N

Nemeh, Issam, 104-10, 130
Nemeh, Kathy, 105, 109

O

ORU (Oral Roberts University), 130
Osler, William, 79-81, 89, 118

P

PBL (problem-based learning), 19
physicians, 10-11, 13-15, 20, 29, 33, 50, 53, 74, 76, 78, 80-82, 84, 86, 97, 100, 108, 110, 115-17, 120-21, 124, 126, 130
PPCSA (Purdue Pharmacy Christian Student Association), 48-49, 58, 62, 64
Purdue Pharmacy Christian Student Association (PPCSA), 48-49, 58, 62

S

Schweitzer, Albert, 81, 89-90
SerVaas, Beurt, 33-34
Siegel, Bernie, 79, 88
spirituality, 1, 3, 15-16, 35, 55, 62, 73, 113

T

Tacker, Willis, 36, 115
TBL (team-based learning), 19
Tierney, Josh, 119, 121-22
Trenton, 66
Turek, John, 39, 49, 59-60, 62

V

Valley Forge, 66

W

Wells, Joseph, 98
Wigglesworth, Smith, 50-52

www.ingramcontent.com/pod-product-compliance
Lightning Source LLC
Chambersburg PA
CBHW061127070526
44584CB00033B/4243